Functional Rhinoplasty

Editor

BENJAMIN C. MARCUS

FACIAL PLASTIC SURGERY CLINICS OF NORTH AMERICA

www.facialplastic.theclinics.com

Consulting Editor
J. REGAN THOMAS

May 2017 • Volume 25 • Number 2

ELSEVIER

1600 John F. Kennedy Boulevard • Suite 1800 • Philadelphia, Pennsylvania, 19103-2899

http://www.theclinics.com

FACIAL PLASTIC SURGERY CLINICS OF NORTH AMERICA Volume 25, Number 2
May 2017 ISSN 1064-7406, ISBN-13: 978-0-323-52838-2

Editor: Jessica McCool
Developmental Editor: Alison Swety

Facial Plastic Surgery Clinics of North America (ISSN 1064-7406) is published quarterly by Elsevier Inc., 360 Park Avenue South, New York, NY 10010-1710. Months of issue are February, May, August, and November. Business and Editorial Offices: 1600 John F. Kennedy Blvd., Suite 1800, Philadelphia, PA 19103-2899. Periodicals postage paid at New York, NY, and additional mailing offices. Subscription prices are $390.00 per year (US individuals), $592.00 per year (US institutions), $445.00 per year (Canadian individuals), $737.00 per year (Canadian institutions), $535.00 per year (foreign individuals), $737.00 per year (foreign institutions), $100.00 per year (US students), and $255.00 per year (foreign students). Foreign air speed delivery is included in all *Clinics* subscription prices. All prices are subject to change without notice. POSTMASTER: Send address changes to *Facial Plastic Surgery Clinics*, Elsevier Health Sciences Division, Subscription Customer Service, 3251 Riverport Lane, Maryland Heights, MO 63043. **Customer service: 1-800-654-2452 (US and Canada); 1-314-447-8871 (outside US and Canada); Fax: 314-447-8029; E-mail: journalscustomerservice-usa@elsevier.com (for print support); journalsonlinesupport-usa@elsevier.com (for online support).**

Reprints. For copies of 100 or more of articles in this publication, please contact the Commercial Reprints Department, Elsevier Inc., 360 Park Avenue South, New York, NY 10010-1710. Tel.: 212-633-3874; Fax: 212-633-3820; E-mail: reprints@elsevier.com.

Facial Plastic Surgery Clinics of North America is covered in *MEDLINE/PubMed* (*Index Medicus*).

Printed in the United States of America.

Contributors

CONSULTING EDITOR

J. REGAN THOMAS, MD, FACS
Professor and Chairman, Department of
Otolaryngology, University of Illinois at
Chicago, Chicago, Illinois

EDITOR

BENJAMIN C. MARCUS, MD
Director of Facial Plastic Surgery, University of
Wisconsin–Madison, Madison, Wisconsin

AUTHORS

ERDINC CEKIC, MD
Department of Otorhinolaryngology–Head
and Neck Surgery, Luttiye Nuri Burat State
Hospital, Sultangazi, Istanbul, Turkey

RAJ DEDHIA, MD
Department of Otolaryngology–Head and Neck
Surgery, UC Davis Medical Center,
Sacramento, California

DREW DEL TORO, BSc
Department of Otolaryngology–Head and Neck
Surgery, UC Davis Medical Center,
Sacramento, California

BRIAN W. DOWNS, MD, FACS
Assistant Professor, Department of
Otolaryngology, Wake Forest Baptist Health,
Winston–Salem, North Carolina

OREN FRIEDMAN, MD
Associate Professor, Clinical
Otorhinolaryngology–Head and Neck
Surgery; Director, Facial Plastic Surgery,
University of Pennsylvania, Philadelphia,
Pennsylvania

GUILHERME J.M. GARCIA, PhD
Assistant Professor, Department of
Otolaryngology and Communication Sciences,
Medical College of Wisconsin; Department of
Biomedical Engineering, Marquette University
and the Medical College of Wisconsin,
Milwaukee, Wisconsin

CEREN GUNEL, MD
Associate Professor, Department of
Otorhinolaryngology–Head and Neck Surgery,
Faculty of Medicine, Adnan Menderes
University, Aydin, Turkey

GRANT S. HAMILTON III, MD
Consultant, Assistant Professor, Department
of Otorhinolaryngology, Mayo Clinic,
Rochester, Minnesota

PETER HILGER, MD, FACS
Professor, Facial Plastic and Reconstructive
Surgery, University of Minnesota, Minneapolis,
Minnesota

TSUNG-YEN HSIEH, MD
Department of Otolaryngology–Head and Neck
Surgery, UC Davis Medical Center,
Sacramento, California

MATTHEW D. JOHNSON, MD
Assistant Professor, Facial Plastic and
Reconstructive Surgery, Division of
Otolaryngology–Head and Neck Surgery,
Southern Illinois University School of Medicine,
Springfield, Illinois

DAVID W. KIM, MD
Division of Facial Plastic and Reconstructive
Surgery, Department of Otolaryngology–Head
and Neck Surgery, University of California,
San Francisco; Private Practice, Facial Plastic
and Reconstructive Surgery, San Francisco,
California

SAM P. MOST, MD
Chief, Division of Facial Plastic and
Reconstructive Surgery; Professor,
Department of Otolaryngology–Head and Neck
Surgery, Stanford University School of
Medicine, Palo Alto, California

JEFFREY S. MOYER, MD
Division of Facial Plastic and Reconstructive
Surgery, Department of Otolaryngology–Head
and Neck Surgery, University of Michigan,
Ann Arbor, Michigan; Center for Facial
Cosmetic Surgery, Livonia, Michigan

SAHAR NADIMI, MD
Department of Otolaryngology–Head and Neck
Surgery, Loyola University Medical Center,
Maywood, Illinois; Private Practice, Facial
Plastic and Reconstructive Surgery, Oakbrook
Terrace, Illinois

SACHIN S. PAWAR, MD
Assistant Professor, Department of
Otolaryngology and Communication Sciences,
Medical College of Wisconsin, Milwaukee,
Wisconsin

JOHN S. RHEE, MD, MPH
Professor and Chairman, Department of
Otolaryngology and Communication Sciences,
Medical College of Wisconsin, Milwaukee,
Wisconsin

JON ROBITSCHEK, MD
Facial Plastics Fellow, University of Minnesota,
Minneapolis, Minnesota

ANDREW J. ROSKO, MD
Division of Facial Plastic and Reconstructive
Surgery, Department of Otolaryngology–Head
and Neck Surgery, University of Michigan,
Ann Arbor, Michigan

SHANNON F. RUDY, MD
Resident, Department of Otolaryngology–Head
and Neck Surgery, Stanford University School
of Medicine, Palo Alto, California

JUSTIN C. SOWDER, MD
Division of Otolaryngology–Head and Neck
Surgery, University of Utah School of Medicine,
Salt Lake City, Utah

ANDREW J. THOMAS, MD
Division of Otolaryngology–Head and Neck
Surgery, University of Utah School of Medicine,
Salt Lake City, Utah

TRAVIS T. TOLLEFSON, MD, MPH, FACS
Professor and Director, Facial Plastic and
Reconstructive Surgery, Department of
Otolaryngology–Head and Neck Surgery, UC
Davis Medical Center, Sacramento, California

KYLE K. VANKOEVERING, MD
Division of Facial Plastic and Reconstructive
Surgery, Department of Otolaryngology–Head
and Neck Surgery, University of Michigan,
Ann Arbor, Michigan

PRESTON DANIEL WARD, MD
Division of Otolaryngology–Head and Neck
Surgery, University of Utah School of Medicine,
Salt Lake City, Utah

Contents

Reduction rhinoplasty techniques include maneuvers that weaken the nasal osseo-cartilaginous framework. The structurally compromised anatomy remaining after reductive surgery may be left with inadequate strength to withstand postoperative contractile forces. Significant aesthetic and functional deformities requiring revision rhinoplasty may develop. This article reviews common causes of nasal obstruction after primary rhinoplasty. The discussion of etiology is based on both the anatomic description of nasal subsites (middle vault and lateral walls) as well as an explanation of why certain techniques lead to functional problems in these areas. Revision rhinoplasty techniques for correcting these problems are discussed in detail.

Advances in computer modeling and simulation technologies have the potential to provide facial plastic surgeons with information and tools that can aid in patient-specific surgical planning for rhinoplasty. Finite element modeling and computational fluid dynamics are modeling technologies that have been applied to the nose to study structural biomechanics and nasal airflow. Combining these technologies with patient-specific imaging data and symptom measures has the potential to alter the future landscape of nasal surgery.

FACIAL PLASTIC SURGERY CLINICS OF NORTH AMERICA

RELATED INTEREST

Clinics in Plastic Surgery, January 2016 (Vol. 43, No. 1)
Rhinoplasty: A Multispecialty Approach
Babak Azizzadeh, *Editor*
Available at: http://www.plasticsurgery.theclinics.com

THE CLINICS ARE AVAILABLE ONLINE!
Access your subscription at:
www.theclinics.com

Preface
Crafting a Functional Nose

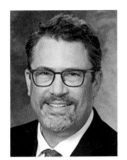

Benjamin C. Marcus, MD
Editor

This issue on functional rhinoplasty provides key insights into the complex world of reconstructive rhinoplasty. We have assembled an all-star panel of authors who have shared their key insights for successful surgery. The full spectrum of clinical situations is investigated in detail. Topics from advanced septoplasty to cleft care are well described. We also offer cutting-edge insights into the latest techniques and technologies for evaluating functional nasal surgery. We hope that you enjoy this critical update on functional nasal surgery and incorporate the insights into your own clinical practice.

Benjamin C. Marcus, MD
University of Wisconsin–Madison
K4/7 Clinical Science Center
600 Highland Avenue
Madison, WI 53792-7375, USA

E-mail address:
marcus@surgery.wisc.edu

Facial Plast Surg Clin N Am 25 (2017) ix
http://dx.doi.org/10.1016/j.fsc.2017.02.001
1064-7406/17/© 2017 Published by Elsevier Inc.

Essential Anatomy and Evaluation for Functional Rhinoplasty

Justin C. Sowder, MD, Andrew J. Thomas, MD,
Preston Daniel Ward, MD*

KEYWORDS

- Rhinoplasty • Functional • Nasal anatomy • Nasal obstruction • Subjective evaluation
- Objective measurements

KEY POINTS

- Successful correction of nasal obstruction requires identification of the precise anatomic cause and a comprehensive understanding of the relationships between surface aesthetics, underlying structural anatomy, and functional components of the nose.
- Subjective evaluation of a patient with nasal obstruction should include systematic examination of the nasal-facial aesthetics with external evaluation, including visual inspection, palpation, and photodocumentation, as well as intranasal examination, including an assessment of nasal valve function.
- Patient-specific quality of life instruments, such as the Nasal Obstruction Symptom Evaluation and visual analog scale, are useful tools to help quantify the degree of nasal obstruction both before and after surgery.
- Several tools have been developed for the objective assessment of nasal obstruction; however, most have not gained widespread use outside of the research setting.

INTRODUCTION

The primary responsibilities of the nose include heating, humidifying, and filtering inspired air before reaching the larynx, trachea, and lungs. This is accomplished via a balance of laminar and turbulent airflow. The laminar flow is responsible for the transmission of air toward the lungs and the turbulent flow, which is related directly to airway resistance, is responsible for the inspired air contacting the nasal mucosa and exchanging molecules to warm and humidify it.[1] When this normally unconscious action is compromised, nasal breathing may become a source of significant distress and decreased quality of life. Nasal obstruction, which may have many different causes, is a common problem and results from a complex interaction of static and dynamic forces on the nasal mucosa and bony-cartilaginous structure of the nose.[2] Before surgically correcting nasal obstruction, the precise anatomic cause must be identified. The surgeon must have a comprehensive understanding of the surface aesthetics, underlying structural anatomy, and functional components of the nose and how they are all linked.[3] The purpose of this article is to highlight the key anatomic structures involved in nasal obstruction and functional rhinoplasty, as well as discuss the diagnostic techniques at the surgeon's disposal to ensure the proper diagnosis is made.

Division of Otolaryngology – Head and Neck Surgery, University of Utah School of Medicine, Salt Lake City, UT 84132, USA
* Corresponding author. Facial Plastic & Reconstructive Surgery, Division of Otolaryngology – Head and Neck Surgery, Ward MD Form Medical, University of Utah School of Medicine, 6322 S 3000 E.Suite 170, Salt Lake City, UT 84132.
E-mail address: doctor@formmedspa.com

Facial Plast Surg Clin N Am 25 (2017) 141–160
http://dx.doi.org/10.1016/j.fsc.2016.12.001
1064-7406/17/

FUNCTIONAL ANATOMY
Bony Pyramid

The bony framework of the nose is pyramidal in shape. It is made up of paired nasal bones that articulate with the frontal bone cephalically and the paired upper lateral cartilages (ULCs) caudally. The confluence of nasal bones, ULCs, and the bony (perpendicular plate of the ethmoid bone) and cartilaginous nasal septum, appropriately known as the keystone area, is critical for midvault support and stability of the nose.[4,5] The nasal bones articulate with the frontal process of the maxilla laterally, and fuse at the midline. They are approximately 25 mm in length, on average, and progressively thin as they approach their inferior confluence with the ULCs.[6] The bony external opening of nasal cavity, the pyriform aperture, is made up of the nasal and frontal bones superiorly and laterally and the maxilla inferiorly. The maxillary crest articulates with the quadrangular cartilage anteriorly and the vomer posteriorly. The perpendicular plate of the ethmoid bone attaches to the cribriform plate cranially and the vomer caudally (**Fig. 1**).

Cartilaginous Pyramid

The cartilaginous nasal pyramid is made up of the cartilaginous nasal septum (or quadrangular cartilage) and the ULCs. They form a T-shape, with the angle formed between the septum and ULCs increasing with cephalad progression from approximately 15° at the internal nasal valve (INV) to 80° at the keystone area.[7] The cartilaginous septum connects caudally with the anterior nasal spine, maxillary crest, and vomer, and freely connects with the columella. The connection with the anterior nasal spine involves collagenous decussating fibers. If these are disrupted during septoplasty, reconstruction is essential to prevent destabilization of the septum.[7] Cranially, the cartilaginous septum connects with the ULCs and its dorsal attachment is the perpendicular plate of the ethmoid bone. The cartilaginous septum ranges from 2 to 4 mm in thickness, and is thicker anteriorly, posteriorly, and at its junction with the ULCs and maxillary crest.[8]

The ULCs are connected cranially with the nasal bones, underlapping them by 1 to 2 mm, and the cartilaginous septum medially along their cephalic

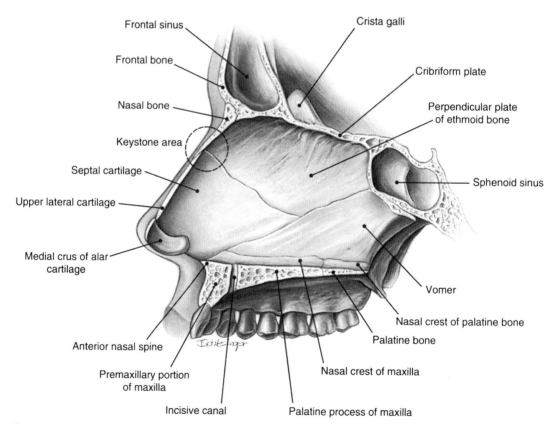

Fig. 1. Lateral view of the left side of the nasal septum. (*From* Oneal RM, Beil RJ. Surgical anatomy of the nose. Clin Plast Surg 2010;37:206; with permission.)

two-thirds. As they extend inferiorly, they flare away from the septum.[9] The ULCs are free of skeletal support laterally but are connected dorsally and laterally with soft tissue. They connect caudally with the cranial margin of the lower lateral cartilages (LLCs) at the scroll region, which is vital in providing nasal tip support (**Fig. 2**). Several small, sesamoid cartilages are found throughout the connective tissue between the ULCs and LLCs (**Figs. 3 and 4**).

Lower Lateral Cartilages

The LLCs (or alar cartilages) are paired cartilages that form the structural component of the nostrils and are the major component of the nasal tip. Each is composed of a medial, intermediate (middle), and lateral crus. The medial crus has a footplate, which attaches to the septal cartilage and is a major source of tip support, and a columellar portion. The medial crus curves and transitions to the intermediate crus at the columellar break point. The intermediate crus is made up of a lobular segment, which is camouflaged by soft tissue and a domal segment, which is responsible for the tip-defining points.[10] The paired intermediate crura are attached to each other via the interdomal ligament. The LLC curves superiorly and forms the lateral crus, which is responsible for determining

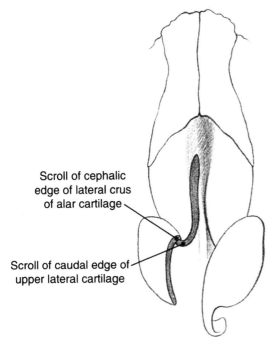

Scroll of cephalic
edge of lateral crus
of alar cartilage

Scroll of caudal edge of
upper lateral cartilage

Fig. 2. Nasal skeleton: frontal view. Note the cut-away section of the right upper and LLCs revealing the scroll region. (*From* Oneal RM, Beil RJ. Surgical anatomy of the nose. Clin Plast Surg 2010;37:201; with permission.)

alar shape. It varies in size (16–30 mm long and 6–16 mm high) and shape (convex, concave, or a combination).[7] The lateral crus is where the caudal LLC and cranial ULC overlap and articulate, forming the scroll area.[11] The posterior border here is attached to the frontal process of the maxilla by dense fibrous tissue and several minor cartilages.[12] Because the lateral crus of the cartilage is angled 45° cephalically, the LLCs only provide support to the medial half of the nasal ala (**Fig. 5**).[13,14]

Lobule

The lobule is composed of the 2 LLCs, connective and fatty tissue, and muscles. It is covered with thick skin and sebaceous glands. The surface anatomy of the lobule is complex and is divided into 5 subunits: the tip, alae, columella, nostril, and vestibule. The tip comprises the supratip, the tip-defining points, and the infratip lobule. The alae are the lateral nasal walls, and are structurally composed of skin, muscles, and the lateral crura of the LLC.

Specific mention should be made regarding the mechanisms of nasal tip support, which are traditionally divided into major and minor (**Box 1**). When performing rhinoplasty, manipulation of any of these mechanisms should be considered carefully to prevent postoperative tip ptosis and resulting nasal obstruction. The tripod theory of nasal tip support, proposed by Anderson[15] in 1968, has become widely accepted by most rhinoplasty surgeons. In this model, the lateral crus of each LLC is described as 2 legs joining the combined medial crura to form a tripod, with the base attached to the frontal plane of the face (**Fig. 6**). Although simplistic, it helps the surgeon visualize how altering either the length or the position of the legs of the tripod will affect tip position. A modification in the tripod theory is the cantilever model proposed by Westreich and Lawson.[16] This model takes into account the elastic potential energy stored in the nasal tip cartilages, as well as the forces from the bony support structures of the face and nose that balance this energy.[17] The surgeon must understand how these forces act on each other to effectively manipulate the nasal tip.

The Nasal Valves

The nose itself is an active resistor to nasal airflow. As one inspires, negative pressure forces air through the nasal cavity. The 2 areas responsible for most upper airway resistance are the external and INVs, with the INV being the major flow-limiting segment.[18] When either of these areas is statically narrow, whether the cause is idiopathic,

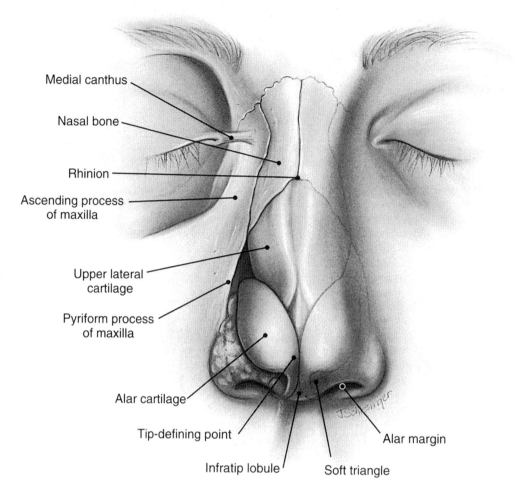

Medial canthus

Nasal bone

Rhinion

Ascending process
of maxilla

Upper lateral
cartilage

Pyriform process
of maxilla

Alar cartilage

Tip-defining point

Infratip lobule

Alar margin

Soft triangle

Fig. 3. Frontal view of nose. (*From* Oneal RM, Beil RJ. Surgical anatomy of the nose. Clin Plast Surg 2010;37: 192; with permission.)

traumatic, or iatrogenic, nasal obstruction results. As air flows through these narrower areas, dynamic valve collapse may also occur. As Poiseuille's law states, resistance is inversely proportional to radius to the fourth power. As air flows through these narrow portions of the nasal passage, the velocity increases and intraluminal pressure decreases, consistent with Bernoulli's principle. This drop in pressure can cause collapse, resulting in a cessation of airflow.[19] Properly functioning nasal valves are a chief determinant of a successful functional rhinoplasty.

External Nasal Valve

The external nasal valve (ENV) is delineated by the alar crease of the nostril superiorly and laterally, by the medial crus of the LLC medially, and the nasal spine and soft tissues overlying the nasal floor inferiorly.[20] ENV obstruction can be static from tip ptosis, vestibular scarring, or stenosis. It may

also be dynamic, due to weak nasal musculature or a weak or malpositioned lateral crus of the LLC.[21] There is also a considerable amount of structural support of the ENV derived from the alar musculature, which forms a sphincter along the nasal inlet (see later discussion).[22]

Internal Nasal Valve

The INV represents the area bordered by the nasal septum medially, the caudal edge of the ULC superolaterally, the head of the inferior turbinate inferolaterally, and the nasal floor inferiorly (**Fig. 7**). The INV is the main source of airflow resistance in the upper airway. The angle between the septum and the ULC should measure 10° to 15° in the nose of a person of white ethnicity. This angle is typically more obtuse in non-whites, resulting in less INV collapse.[23] There are 4 functional components of the INV, as described by Cole,[24] and abnormalities in any can result in nasal

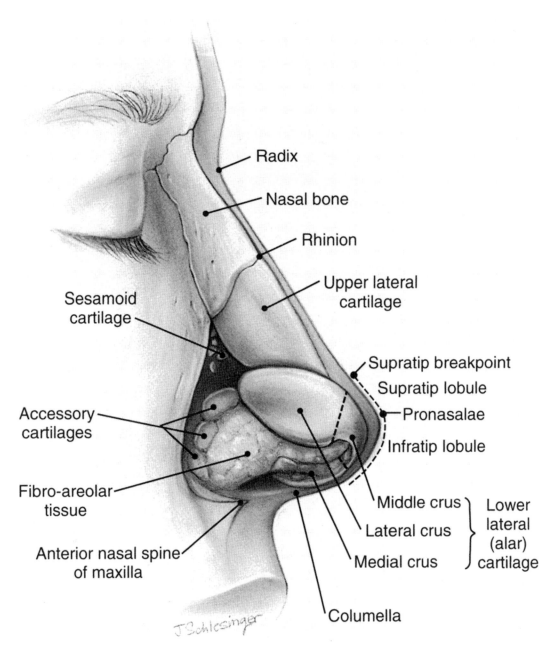

Fig. 4. Right lateral view of nose. (*From* Oneal RM, Beil RJ. Surgical anatomy of the nose. Clin Plast Surg 2010;37:192; with permission.)

obstruction (**Table 1**). Static INV dysfunction can result from medialized ULCs, whether idiopathic or due to failure to stabilize the ULC following reduction rhinoplasty. Similarly, an hourglass deformity can result if the ULCs fall into the nasal cavity following hump reduction.[1] Patients with short nasal bones, thin skin, and an overprojected and narrow middle vault, known as the narrow nose syndrome, are also prone to INV narrowing and nasal obstruction.[25] A caudal septal deformity

or hypertrophic inferior turbinates (see later discussion) can also decrease the INV area.

Inferior Turbinates

The inferior turbinate is made up a long, thin, curled bone that attaches to the lateral nasal wall and extends medial into the nasal cavity. It is covered by a mucosal layer made up of pseudostratified columnar ciliated respiratory epithelium.

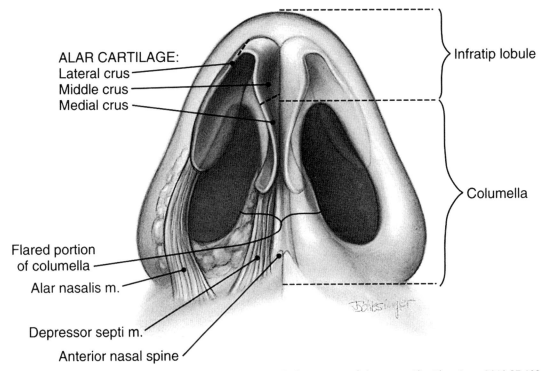

ALAR CARTILAGE:
Lateral crus
Middle crus
Medial crus

Infratip lobule

Columella

Flared portion
of columella
Alar nasalis m.

Depressor septi m.
Anterior nasal spine

Fig. 5. Basal view of nose. (*From* Oneal RM, Beil RJ. Surgical anatomy of the nose. Clin Plast Surg 2010;37:192; with permission.)

Box 1
Major and minor tip support mechanisms

Major

1. Size, shape, and resilience of the medial and lateral crura
2. Medial crural footplate attachment to the caudal border of the quadrangular cartilage
3. Attachment of the upper lateral cartilages (caudal border) to the alar cartilages (cephalic border)

Minor

1. The ligamentous sling spanning the paired domes of the alar cartilages (interdomal ligament)
2. The cartilaginous dorsal septum
3. The sesamoid complex supporting the connection of the lateral crura to the piriform aperture
4. The attachment of the alar cartilage to the overlying skin and musculature (skin and soft-tissue envelope)
5. The nasal spine
6. The membranous septum

Adapted from Gassner HG, Sherris DA, Friedman O. Rhinology in rhinoplasty. In: Papel I, editor. Facial plastic and reconstructive surgery. New York: Thieme; 2009. p. 492.

Well-developed erectile tissue is located along the inferior turbinate, which is composed of venous sinusoids that drain the capillary system of the nasal mucosa.[2] The inferior turbinate has a large surface area and is largely responsible for the warming, humidifying, and filtering of inspired air, as well as directing it toward the nasopharynx.[26] The head of the inferior turbinate is the inferolateral border of the INV. When it becomes congested it can decrease the cross-sectional area of the valve, resulting in obstructed breathing. Selective submucous resection and lateralization can help to alleviate nasal obstruction; however, this should be done judiciously because over-resection can lead to atrophic rhinitis.[27]

Skin and Soft Tissue Envelope

The soft tissue covering of the osseocartilaginous structure of the nose is made up of skin, subcutaneous tissues, and muscle, and serves as a source of minor nasal tip support. The nasal skin varies in thickness by location on the nose. It is generally thicker over the nasofrontal angle, thins as it approaches the rhinion, where it is thinnest, and then thickens again as it approaches the supratip, tip, and nasal ala, where it is thickest. The skin thins again along the alar margin and columella. The thicker skin is in part due to a higher density of sebaceous glands, particularly at the

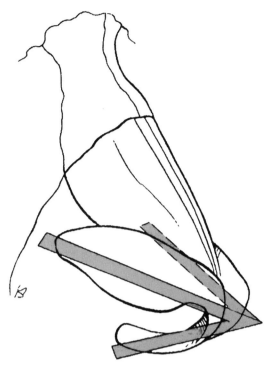

Fig. 6. Tripod concept of nasal tip cartilages. (*From* Oneal RM, Beil RJ. Surgical anatomy of the nose. Clin Plast Surg 2010;37:199; with permission.)

nasal tip. Non-white patients typically have thicker skin with increased sebaceous glands, which can hide small surgical imperfections but has a higher incidence of postoperative fibrosis and supratip deformities.[27,28] Conversely, thinner skin is less forgiving and great care must be taken when manipulating the underlying skeleton to ensure aesthetically pleasing results.

The soft tissue envelope of the nose is composed of 4 distinct layers.[29] The superficial fatty layer is tightly adherent to the overlying

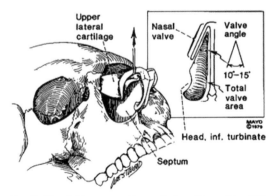

Fig. 7. The INV area and boundaries. (*From* Kim DW, Rodriguez-Bruno K. Functional rhinoplasty. Facial Plast Surg Clin North Am 2009;17(1):118; with permission.)

Table 1 The 4 functional components of the nasal valve	
Segment	**Description**
I	INV angle
II	Bony piriform aperture
III	Head of the inferior turbinate
IV	Erectile body of the septum

Segments I and II represent the structural segments, and segments III and IV the mucovascular segments.
    Adapted from Cole P. The four components of the nasal valve. Am J Rhinol 2003;17:108–9.

dermis. Deep to this is the fibromuscular layer, or superficial musculoaponeurotic system (SMAS), which contains the nasal musculature. The next deepest layer is the deep fatty layer, which overlies the perichondrial-periosteal layer that is tightly adherent to the osseocartilaginous components. The avascular plane of dissection used to deglove the nose during open rhinoplasty lies between the fibromuscular and perichondrial-periosteal layers so as to avoid disrupting the SMAS and neurovascular structures.[10]

Muscles

The nasal musculature is ensheathed in the SMAS layer, whose function is to distribute the tensile forces of the nasal musculature and to provide a sling for the mimetic muscles to counteract against.[27] Originally described by Mitz and Peyronie,[30] the nasal SMAS layer covers the external nose from the glabella to the caudal margin of the nostrils and is continuous with the facial SMAS, the platysma, and the galea aponeurosis.[31] Failure to respect the SMAS layer when degloving the nose can lead to retraction of the layer if transected, which can result in scarring of the dermis to the underlying osseocartilaginous components. The nasal musculature that is ensheathed within the SMAS layer is broken down into 4 groups by Griesman[11]: the elevators, the depressors, the minor dilator, and the compressors, as seen in **Fig. 8** and **Table 2**. These muscles have implications on both the aesthetic and functional aspects of rhinoplasty. For example, overactivity of the depressors can cause tip ptosis, and weak or poorly developed dilators can lead to external valve collapse, both of which result in nasal obstruction.

Blood Supply

Most of the nasal vasculature and lymphatics are found within or slightly superficial to the nasal SMAS layer.[32] The arterial supply of the external nose comes from the external carotid artery, via

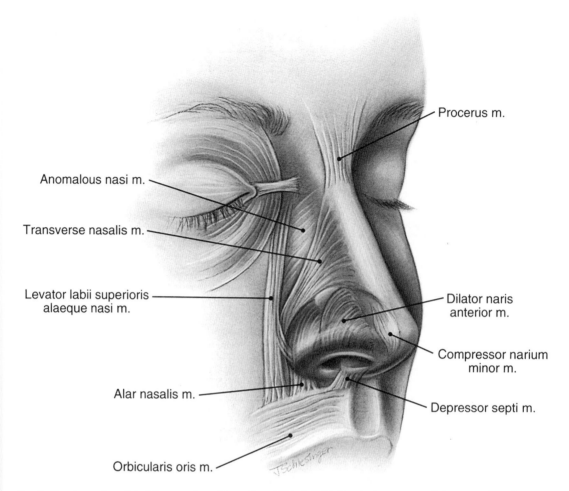

Anomalous nasi m.

Transverse nasalis m.

Levator labii superioris alaeque nasi m.

Alar nasalis m.

Orbicularis oris m.

Procerus m.

Dilator naris anterior m.

Compressor narium minor m.

Depressor septi m.

Fig. 8. Nasal muscles of facial expression. (*From* Oneal RM, Beil RJ. Surgical anatomy of the nose. Clin Plast Surg 2010;37:193; with permission.)

Table 2
Nasal muscle groups by action

	Muscles	Action
Elevators	Procerus Levator labii superioris alaeque nasi Anomalous nasi	Shorten nose Dilate nostrils
Depressors	Alar portion of nasalis (dilator naris posterior) Depressor septi	Lengthen nose Dilate nostrils
Minor dilator	Dilator naris anterior	Dilate nostrils
Compressors	Transverse portion of Nasalis Compressor narium minor	Lengthen nose Narrow nostrils

the facial and infraorbital branches, and the internal carotid artery, via the anterior ethmoid branch of the ophthalmic artery (**Fig. 9**). The vascular supply of the internal nose is supplied by the anterior and posterior ethmoid arteries, the septal branch of the superior labial artery, and the sphenopalatine branch of the internal maxillary artery, which converge in Kiesselbach plexus (**Figs. 10** and **11**). Venous drainage of the nose is via similarly named veins that accompany the arteries, which drain via the facial vein to the pterygoid plexus and the ophthalmic veins to the cavernous sinus.[29] Notably, the veins are without valves, and infections of the nose can spread intracranially if left untreated.

Nerves

The sensory innervation of the nose is via the ophthalmic (V1) and maxillary (V2) divisions of the

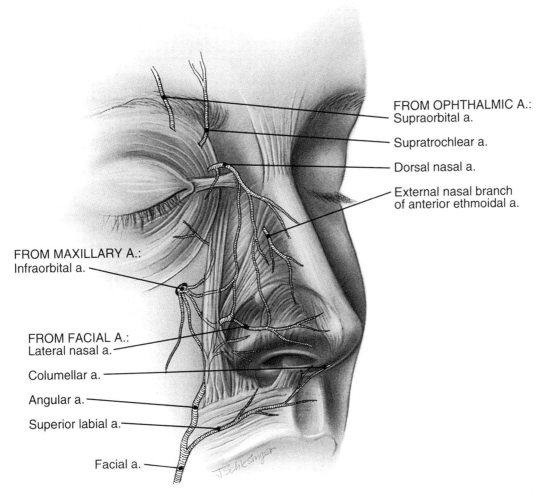

FROM OPHTHALMIC A.:
Supraorbital a.

Supratrochlear a.

Dorsal nasal a.

External nasal branch
of anterior ethmoidal a.

FROM MAXILLARY A.:
Infraorbital a.

FROM FACIAL A.:
Lateral nasal a.

Columellar a.

Angular a.

Superior labial a.

Facial a.

Fig. 9. Arterial blood supply of the external nose. (*From* Oneal RM, Beil RJ. Surgical anatomy of the nose. Clin Plast Surg 2010;37:193; with permission.)

trigeminal nerve. The external innervation is supplied by the supratrochlear, infratrochlear, and external nasal branch of the anterior ethmoidal nerves from V1, and the infraorbital nerve branch from V2 (**Fig. 12**). Internally, the septum is innervated by the medial internal nasal branch of the anterior ethmoidal nerve (V1) and the nasopalatine nerve (V2) (**Fig. 13**). The lateral nasal walls are innervated by the lateral internal nasal branch of the anterior ethmoidal nerve (V1) and the greater and lesser palatine nerves (V2) (**Fig. 14**). The zygomatico-temporal branch of the facial nerve innervates all of the nasal musculature.

PATIENT EVALUATION
Subjective Evaluation

Nasal-facial analysis
The primary goal of functional rhinoplasty is to relieve nasal obstruction without negatively

affecting nasal aesthetics. To do so, one must understand how the structures of the face relate to each other proportionally. The face should be evaluated systematically in multiple views: frontal, profile (lateral), oblique, and base. Specific nasal deformities that can be identified on each view are listed in **Table 3**. The face is classically divided into horizontal thirds and vertical fifths in the frontal view to assess for facial balance. The width of the alar base makes up the middle fifth, equal to the intercanthal width. The width of the base of the bony sidewall of the nose is roughly 75% the width of the alar base.[33] To help assess for symmetry, a gently curving line can be drawn from the medial brow to the ipsilateral nasal tip-defining point, making the brow-tip aesthetic line (**Fig. 15**).[34] An underprojected tip or narrowed middle third can result in irregularities in the contour of this line. Dorsal deviation is readily apparent when a vertical line is drawn from the menton to the

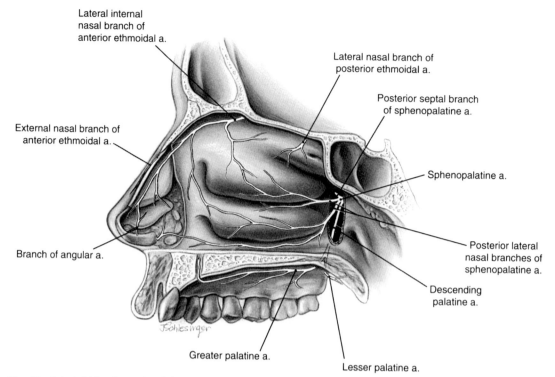

Lateral internal nasal branch of anterior ethmoidal a.

Lateral nasal branch of posterior ethmoidal a.

Posterior septal branch of sphenopalatine a.

External nasal branch of anterior ethmoidal a.

Sphenopalatine a.

Branch of angular a.

Posterior lateral nasal branches of sphenopalatine a.

Descending palatine a.

Greater palatine a.

Lesser palatine a.

Fig. 10. Arterial blood supply of the right lateral nasal wall. (*From* Oneal RM, Beil RJ. Surgical anatomy of the nose. Clin Plast Surg 2010;37:209; with permission.)

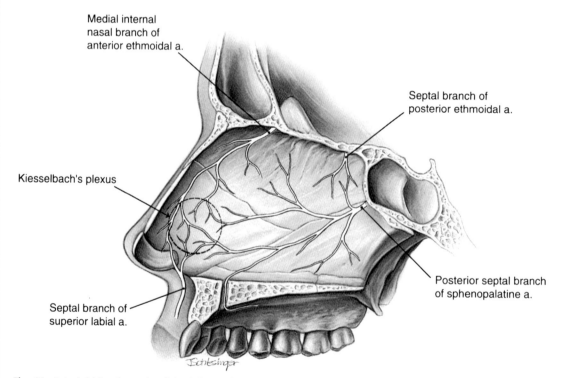

Medial internal nasal branch of anterior ethmoidal a.

Septal branch of posterior ethmoidal a.

Kiesselbach's plexus

Posterior septal branch of sphenopalatine a.

Septal branch of superior labial a.

Fig. 11. Arterial blood supply of the left nasal septum. (*From* Oneal RM, Beil RJ. Surgical anatomy of the nose. Clin Plast Surg 2010;37:209; with permission.)

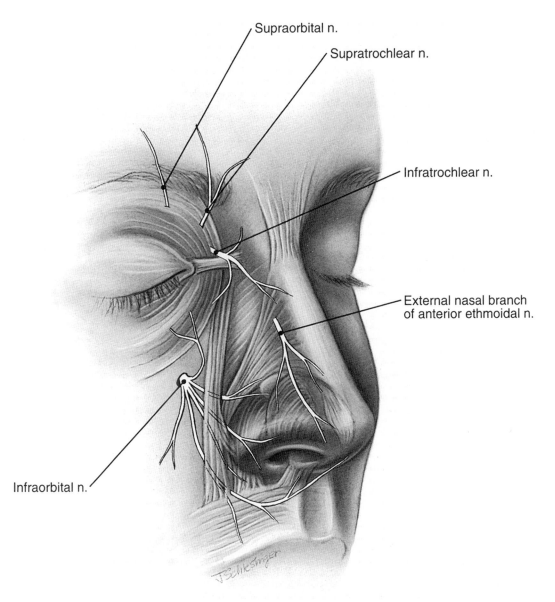

Fig. 12. Sensory nerve supply of the external nose. (*From* Oneal RM, Beil RJ. Surgical anatomy of the nose. Clin Plast Surg 2010;37:194; with permission.)

midglabellar region. A C-shaped deformity occurs when there is an irregularity in the septum or ULCs, and tip deviation may result from aberration of anterior septal angle or LLCs.[35] The anteriormost projection of the intermediate crura forms tip-defining points, which can be identified by light reflection in the frontal view.[36]

When assessing from the profile view, it is important to have the head in the Frankfort horizontal plane. In the Frankfort horizontal plane, a line drawn from the superior external auditory canal through the inferior orbital rim is perpendicular to the floor. Tip projection, rotation, and nasal length are assessed from the lateral view. The nose should make a 3-4-5 right-angled triangle, with nasal projection 60% of the nasal length.[37] The ideal male nasolabial angle is 90° to 95° and the ideal female nasolabial angle is 95° to 115°, whereas the nasofrontal angle is typically from 115° to 130°. The nasal dorsum is best evaluated from the profile view and, ideally, should lie 1 to 2 mm inferior and parallel to a line drawn from the nasion to the nasal tip. The degree of columellar show is also examined and should be between 2 and 4 mm.

The third external view is the base view, which allows for evaluation of nostril size and shape,

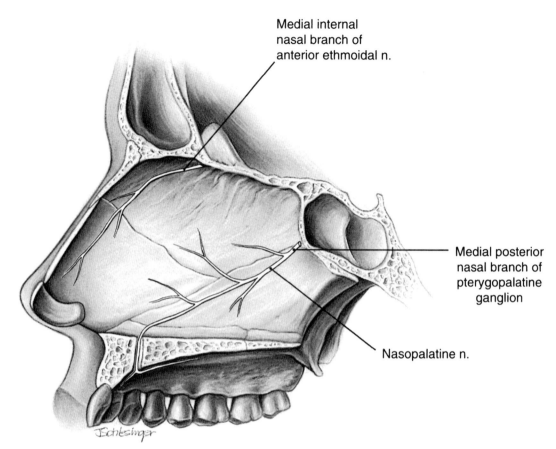

Medial internal
nasal branch of
anterior ethmoidal n.

Medial posterior
nasal branch of
pterygopalatine
ganglion

Nasopalatine n.

Fig. 13. Sensory nerve supply of the left nasal septum. (*From* Oneal RM, Beil RJ. Surgical anatomy of the nose. Clin Plast Surg 2010;37:208; with permission.)

columellar and alar base width, LLC recurvature, and lobule height and contour. On this view, the nose should appear as an isosceles triangle, with a columella-to-lobule ratio of 2:1, although this ranges from 1.3 to 1.5:1 among African Americans, Asians, and Latinos (**Fig. 16**).[33,38–41] If LLC recurvature is present, it must be recognized because tip narrowing in these patients can result in creation of iatrogenic nasal obstruction.[35] The nostrils should be pear-shaped, symmetric, and widest along the nasal sill, with their width being approximately the same as that of the columella. Some surgeons advocate assessing the patient via a helicopter view from above to help assist in evaluating dorsal deviation, nasal bridge and base widths, alar flare, and domal symmetry.[42]

Quality of life measures

Nasal Obstruction Symptom Evaluation The Nasal Obstruction Symptom Evaluation (NOSE) is a validated disease-specific instrument for evaluating nasal obstruction symptom severity.[43] This instrument is grouped into 5 different categories of nasal congestion, nasal blockage, trouble breathing,

trouble sleeping, and inability to get air through the nose during exercise. Each category is scored from 0 to 4 (not a problem to severe problem), and the scores are then scaled to a maximum possible score of 100 by multiplying by 5 (**Table 4**). Scores of 5 to 25 have been classified as mild, 30 to 50 as moderate, 55 to 75 as severe, and 80 to 100 as extreme nasal obstruction.[44] NOSE scores for patients with chronic nasal obstruction, asymptomatic patients, and postoperative nasal obstruction patients have been reported as a mean (SD) of 65 (22), 23 (20), and 15 (17), respectively.[45] The utility of this measure was initially demonstrated when applied to patients undergoing septoplasty, finding a significant statistical and clinical improvement in postoperative NOSE score.[46] Subsequently, significant NOSE score improvement has been demonstrated after addressing other anatomic sites of nasal obstruction, including correction of nasal valve compromise (INV or ENV),[47] specific repair of ENV[48,49] or INV dysfunction alone,[48] and reduction of turbinate hypertrophy.[48] Additional evidence has also supported NOSE score improvement with septoplasty.[48,50]

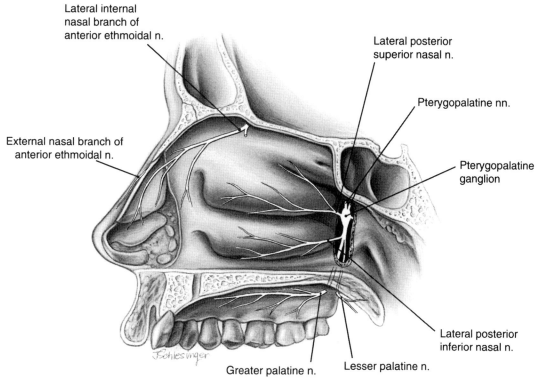

Lateral internal nasal branch of anterior ethmoidal n.

Lateral posterior superior nasal n.

Pterygopalatine nn.

External nasal branch of anterior ethmoidal n.

Pterygopalatine ganglion

Lateral posterior inferior nasal n.

Greater palatine n. Lesser palatine n.

Fig. 14. Sensory nerve supply of the right lateral nasal wall. (*From* Oneal RM, Beil RJ. Surgical anatomy of the nose. Clin Plast Surg 2010;37:208; with permission.)

Table 3
Nasal deformities by view

View	Deformity
Frontal	Inverted V
	Twisted dorsum
	Bifid tip
	Pinched tip
	Parenthetic tip
Lateral	Low or high radix
	Inadequately positioned nasion
	Dorsal hump
	Saddle nose
	Pollybeak
	Underprojection or overprojection
	Alar notching
	Ptotic tip
	Tension nose
Base	Boxy tip
	Bulbous tip
	Bifid tip
	Amorphous tip
	Caudal septal deviation

Adapted from Woodard CR, Park SS. Nasal and facial analysis. Clin Plast Surg 2010;37:183; with permission.

Although the NOSE score has demonstrated utility as an instrument for assessing symptomatic nasal obstruction, a few caveats regarding its use should be considered. First, the NOSE score was designed to compare groups of patients undergoing different treatments and not for use in individual patients. So, although the NOSE score could potentially be helpful to the clinician in quantifying change in nasal obstruction for an individual patient, the instrument was not designed or validated for this purpose. Additionally, the NOSE obstruction-focused questions such as those addressing "obstruction" and "trouble breathing" have demonstrated poor correlation with other disease-specific quality of life measures in patients with chronic rhinosinusitis.[51] This suggests the need to interpret these scores with care in context of treating the true underlying cause of morbidity to the patient. In rhinosinusitis, the underlying inflammatory disease may be the most important element to address and surgery focused on nasal obstruction, without treating inflammatory disease, may improve the NOSE score without clinically relevant improvement in the patient's quality of life.

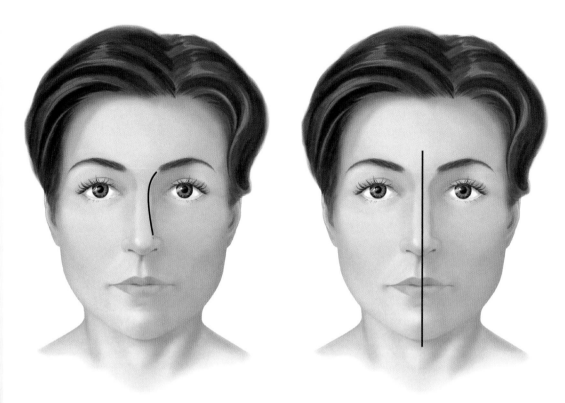

Fig. 15. Brow-tip aesthetic line follows a gentle curve from the medial brow to the nasal tip. (*From* Orten SS, Hilger PA. Facial analysis of the rhinoplasty patient. In Papel ID, editor. Facial plastic and reconstructive surgery. New York: Thieme, 2002; with permission.)

Visual analog scale The visual analog scale (VAS) is a general concept of translating a subjective feeling into a quantifiable numerical rating using a linear scale.[45] This concept is obviously not unique to the evaluation of nasal obstruction but has been applied successfully for this purpose. Patients are asked to rank their degree of nasal obstruction along a graphic linear scale ranging from "none or no obstruction" to "severe or

complete obstruction," which is then converted to a numeric 0 to 10 score. Although the NOSE score and VAS score have demonstrated strong correlation with each other, a key difference between these assessments is that the VAS can be applied separately to each side of the nose.[52] VAS scores have been demonstrated to correlate to preoperative nasal resistance as determined by rhinomanometry for the more obstructed nasal cavity, whereas NOSE scores did not correlate with measured nasal resistance.[52] Similar to the NOSE instrument, significant improvements have been demonstrated in the VAS of nasal obstruction following various methods of functional rhinoplasty with procedures performed in aggregate[48,53] or for isolated procedures addressing the INV, ENV, or septum and turbinates.[48] VAS scores to address chronic nasal obstruction for patients who are afflicted with chronic nasal obstruction, are asymptomatic, or are postoperative from surgery have been reported as a mean (SD) 6.9 (2.3), 2.1 (2.2), and 2.1 (1.6), respectively.[45]

Interalar Distance

1/3

1/3

1/3

Alar-Facial Groove

Nasal Vestibule   Nasal Sill

Nasal Flare

Fig. 16. Basal view of the nose with 2:1 columella to lobule ratio. (*From* Ponsky D, Guyuron B. Alar base disharmonies. Clin Plast Surg 2010;37(2):246; with permission.)

Palpation Gaining an understanding of the dynamics of tissue and support of the nose by palpation is a necessity in the surgical evaluation for

Table 4
Nasal Obstruction Symptom Evaluation instrument

Over the past month, how much of a problem were the following conditions for you?
Please circle the most correct response

	Not a problem	Very mild problem	Moderate problem	Fairly bad problem	Severe problem
1. Nasal congestion or stuffiness	0	1	2	3	4
2. Nasal blockage or obstruction	0	1	2	3	4
3. Trouble breathing through my nose	0	1	2	3	4
4. Trouble sleeping	0	1	2	3	4
5. Unable to get enough air through my nose	0	1	2	3	4

Adapted from Stewart MG, Witsell DL, Smith TL, et al. Development and validation of the Nasal Obstruction Symptom Evaluation (NOSE) scale. Otolaryngol Head Neck Surg 2004;130(2):162; with permission.

rhinoplasty. Small changes observed in the texture or elasticity of skin can dramatically alter surgical technique, approach, and outcomes. The intrinsic strength, size, and support of the septum, ULCs, and LLCs can be easily evaluated by palpation (**Table 5**). The nasal bones should also be palpated to help determine their size and the presence of any bony step-offs.[35]

Cottle and modified Cottle maneuvers One important portion of the subjective nasal examination that cannot be overlooked is the evaluation of the INVs and ENVs. The nasal valves are major contributors to the resistance of nasal airflow.[54,55] Two tests have been commonly used to evaluate the INVs and ENVs, and have been shown to predict outcomes in functional rhinoplasty.[56] The Cottle maneuver is performed by pulling on a patient's cheek in an upward and lateral orientation (**Fig. 17A**). Improved breathing with the Cottle

maneuver has been suggested to implicate valvular collapse, though the finding is nonspecific and improved breathing may similarly result with other causes of obstruction (eg, turbinate hypertrophy or septal deviation). The modified Cottle maneuver involves placing a cotton-tipped applicator in the nose and supporting either the INV or ENV against collapse (**Fig. 17B**). This test is, therefore, more specific than the original Cottle maneuver for evaluating valve dysfunction and can specifically identify which nasal valve is contributing. A positive modified Cottle test has been associated with positive outcomes after addressing the nasal valves surgically. The correlation between preoperative improvement in breathing with support of the INV and postoperative improvement after performing spreader grafts

Table 5
Methods of palpation

Structure	Method to Evaluate
Anterior septal angle	Downward pressure just superior to nasal tip
LLC	Upward pressure on nasal tip
Alar cartilage	Downward pressure on nasal tip with immediate release. Examine recoil.
Septum	Finger and thumb in each vestibule applying central and pulling pressure.

Adapted from Pietro P, Khodaei I, Tasman A. A Guide to the Assessment and Analysis of the Rhinoplasty Patient. Rhinoplasty, The Experts Reference. A. Sclafani. New York: Thieme; 2015. pp. 27–31; with permission.

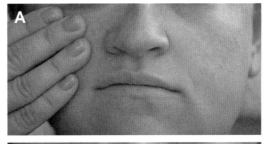
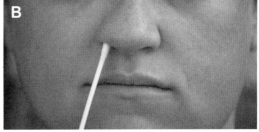

Fig. 17. Cottle (*A*) and modified Cottle (*B*) maneuvers to test for nasal valve dysfunction.

is strong. There is also a moderate correlation between preoperative improvement with ENV support and postoperative improvement with alar batten grafting.[56]

Intranasal examination: anterior rhinoscopy and endoscopy The 3 most common surgical problem areas in a patient with nasal obstruction are the septum, the inferior turbinate, and the lateral nasal wall.[57] Therefore, in the examination of a patient with concerns for nasal obstruction, it is essential to visualize these structures. Anterior rhinoscopy is commonly used to examine the anterior to middle nasal cavity. Use of anterior rhinoscopy can provide details regarding the quality of the anterior nasal mucosa, the size of the inferior turbinates, and whether or not a large anterior septal deviation is present.[58]

In addition to anterior rhinoscopy, many rhinoplasty surgeons recommend the addition of nasal endoscopy as part of the standard examination of patients with nasal obstruction. Not only can it provide better detail of the anterior nasal cavity but one can take photos for review as well. Nasal endoscopy can also help elucidate the posterior nasal cavity and help obtain better appreciation of the pyriform aperture and the choanae. Nasal endoscopy is especially important in patients presenting with unilateral obstruction because many times polyps or tumors in the nasal cavity can present superiorly or posteriorly, and out of view of anterior rhinoscopy.[58]

Whether using anterior rhinoscopy or endoscopy, it is important to evaluate the structures both before and after using decongestant. Before using decongestant, one can appreciate the nasal cavity in its normal state and can obtain better view of turbinate size and general swelling of mucosa, which can contribute significantly to nasal obstruction. After introducing the decongestant, the examination will be removed of any swollen mucosa and can help show the true anatomic cause of obstruction, if present. The combination of examinations can ultimately elucidate all of the contributing factors leading to obstruction in a patient.

Photoanalysis One of the most important steps in surgical planning for rhinoplasty is to reassess the specific anatomy by taking facial photographs. These images can also be useful for discussions with the patient in regard to their unique anatomy and surgical approaches to consider. Standard views include frontal, three-quarter turn, profile, and base (**Fig. 18**A–D). Each specific view helps to examine different contours of the face and nose. Some surgeons have also described the helicopter view as being particularly helpful. This view, which is a photograph from above the patient, provides invaluable information in regard to alar position, general symmetry, and nasal bridge depth (**Fig. 18**E).[59]

OBJECTIVE MEASUREMENTS OF NASAL OBSTRUCTION
Rhinomanometry

Developed in the twentieth century, rhinomanometry involves utilization of a pressure sensor and flow sensor to calibrate the flow of air as a function of pressure for each separate nasal cavity. This technique is performed by occluding 1 naris with a pressure sensor and leaving the contralateral naris open. The patient is then fitted with a mask, which

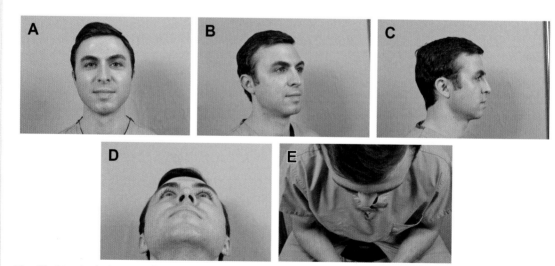

Fig. 18. Standard photographic views include (*A*) frontal, (*B*) three-quarter turn, (*C*) profile, (*D*) base, and (*E*) helicopter.

incorporates a flow sensor, and asked to breathe. The pressure measured on the occluded side is thought to be a good estimation of the pressure in the contralateral nasal cavity. The pressure and flow data are then recorded and converted graphically to be analyzed. Anterior rhinomanometry is most common, although posterior and postnasal modifications to this technique exist. Rhinomanometry has been used to assess outcomes following surgery for nasal obstruction.[60] Although there has been much interest in rhinomanometry, factors that limit its reliability as an objective measurement must be noted, including lack of standardized interpretation of flow graphs and inability to assess dynamic function of the nasal valve.

Acoustic Rhinometry

Created by Hilberg and colleagues,[61] acoustic rhinometry (AR) is an objective measure of nasal cavity function that calculates the cross-sectional area of the nasal cavity as a function of the distance into the nasal cavity from the nasal sill. This measurement is obtained by analyzing local changes in acoustic reflections as soundwaves travel through the nasal cavity. It provides graphical data of the nasal cavity, including volume and changes over time. The graphical data is presented as an area versus distance curve, which results in a W-shape with 2 notches that represent nasal valve constriction and the inferior turbinate, respectively. AR is a static measurement of nasal dimensions. The measurements obtained are affected by the degree of nasal congestion at the time they are taken. Lee and Most[62] recommend obtaining measurements both before and after applying topical decongestants to determine to what degree mucosal hypertrophy is contributing to the patient's nasal obstruction.

Imaging Studies

Computed tomography (CT) and MRI have been used for radiographic assessment of nasal obstruction. CT allows for assessment of the nasal valve angle, which is critical to addressing nasal obstruction. However, measurements depend on the particular view analyzed and the most accurate measurements are described from nontraditional views.[63,64] The nasal base view (NBV) is a view performed in the plane perpendicular to the anterior aspect of the estimated acoustic axis. It has been described as most closely approximating the true measurement of the INV.[64] A significant difference was found between the angle as measured by standard coronal views and the angle measured by the NBV, which more closely approximated classically described ranges of 10° to 15° compared with the

narrower measurements obtained in the coronal plan.[64] Although these measurements obtained using the NBV correlate well with measurements obtained by AR, there are limited studies to validate the reproducibility and utility of this technique.[63] Additionally, measurements of the INV area and angle failed to correlate with the modified Cottle score, demonstrating a lack of significant relationship to the functional outcome of interest for surgical intervention.[65] CT has also been described for evaluating the middle and posterior nasal passage at the level of the osteomeatal unit and the choanae, respectively, for which preoperative NOSE and VAS scores correlate with anatomic features that may be underappreciated by endoscopy and are not well evaluated by AR.[66] Given the limited clinical utility for these CT-based measurements, requirement of reformatting to a nonstandard view for the most accurate measurement and the need to obtain a CT for a patient who may not otherwise require it, routine use of the CT imaging for preoperative planning cannot yet be recommended.

Imaging by CT or MRI can also be used to create 3-dimensional reconstructions, which can then be used to simulate nasal airflow by the method of computational fluid dynamics (CFD). Unilateral nasal airflow anywhere along the nasal airway can be determined to precisely localize impeding anatomic areas. Calculations from these models can determine nasal resistance, as well as heat transfer and humidification. In the example shown in **Fig. 19**, CFD is used to model airflow streamlines and velocity (**Fig. 19**A) as well as wall shear stress (see **Fig. 19**B), in patients with asymptomatic (N1, 2, 3) and symptomatic (S1, 2, 3) nasal septal deviation. In addition to modeling airflow in the present state of the nose, CFD can be used to perform virtual surgery and make predictions about surgical outcomes.[67,68] Advantages compared with rhinomanometry include the ability to measure nasal resistance at normal resting breathing because rhinomanometry requires higher than normal airflow rate with nasal resistance measured over a pressure drop of 150 Pa and to precisely localize unilateral areas of increased nasal resistance.[68] However, there are caveats to this method as well. First, this is a computer simulation, which must make assumptions to satisfy the requirements of the mathematical models and some assumptions may not accurately reflect actual anatomy and physiology (eg, the nasal cavity being considered a fixed and rigid structure).[69] Greater accuracy and utility of this technique is anticipated as the technology continues to improve. Preoperative manipulation of nasal models has shown correlation to

A   **B**

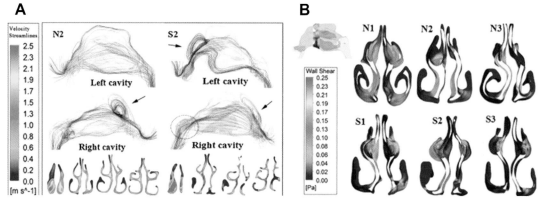

Fig. 19. CFD model of inspiratory air at a flow-rate of 250 mL/s. (*A*) Streamlines and velocity distribution maps are shown for asymptomatic (N2) patients with nasal septum deviation as well as symptomatic patients (S2). The streamlines identify areas of laminar appearing flow as well as vortexes (*arrows* and *dotted ring*) that appeared in front of the middle turbinate and at the nasopharynx. The velocity magnitude distributions reveal higher velocities in the symptomatic patients and greatest velocities in the nasal valve area. (*B*) Wall shear stress is calculated, here focusing on the anterior surface of the middle turbinate in asymptomatic (N1, 2, 3) and symptomatic (S1, 2, 3) patients. Symptomatic patients demonstrate higher shear stress in this example. N, asymptomatic patients; S, symptomatic patients. (*From* Kim SK, Heo GE, Seo A, et al. Correlation between nasal airflow characteristics and clinical relevance of nasal septal deviation to nasal airway obstruction. Respir Physiol Neurobiol 2014;192:99; with permission.)

postoperative results by CFD, though a lack of accuracy has been noted, with surgeon-predicted improvement in airflow and reduction in nasal resistance exceeding postoperative results.[67] Other obvious drawbacks to CFD are additional expense, time, and radiation exposure (for CT-based models, which have better resolution than MRI). Although the cost and time associated with producing these models continues to decrease, the additional expense and imaging must be weighed against the ability to actually improve outcomes, and further work is needed to establish the value of this procedure.[63]

Rhinoresiliography

As previously mentioned, ENV collapse secondary to a ptotic or weak nasal tip can result in nasal obstruction. Rhinoresiliography was developed to objectively measure the tissue resilience and recoil of the nasal tip in relationship to force over distance.[70] In this technique, a transducer is connected to the nasal tip, which can measure force applied (resilience) to tissue and force received from tissue (recoil). The principle is that the force needed to move tissue (resilience) is larger than the recoil from tissue to regain original shape. Objective and normative values for nasal tip resilience and recoil have been gathered to use as controls.[70,71] However, aside from research use in quantification of nasal tip support, the clinical utility of this technique and relationship to rhinoplasty outcomes has not been demonstrated.

SUMMARY

Nasal obstruction is a common problem that results from a complex interaction of static and dynamic forces on the nasal mucosa and bony-cartilaginous structure of the nose. Successful correction of nasal obstruction requires identification of the precise anatomic cause and a comprehensive understanding of how the surface aesthetics, underlying structural anatomy, and functional components of the nose are all linked. Subjective evaluation of the nasal obstruction patient should include systematic examination of the nasal-facial aesthetics with photodocumentation, palpation, intranasal examination, and assessment of nasal valve function. Patient-specific quality of life instruments, such as NOSE and VAS, are useful adjuncts that help quantify the degree of nasal obstruction both before and after surgery. Although several tools have been developed for the objective assessment of nasal obstruction, currently, most have not gained widespread use outside of the research setting.

REFERENCES

1. Ballert JA, Park SS. Functional considerations in revision rhinoplasty. Facial Plast Surg 2008;24: 348–57.
2. Ghosh A, Friedman O. Surgical treatment of nasal obstruction in rhinoplasty. Clin Plast Surg 2016;43: 29–40.

3. Cakir B, Oreroglu AR, Daniel RK. Surface aesthetics and analysis. Clin Plast Surg 2016;43:1–15.

4. Drumheller GW. Topology of the lateral nasal cartilages: the anatomical relationship of the lateral nasal to the greater alar cartilage, lateral crus. Anat Rec 1973;176:321–7.

5. Pitanguy I. Surgical Importance of a Dermocartilaginous Ligament in Bulbous Noses. Plast Reconstr Surg 1965;36:247–53.

6. Wright WK. Surgery of the bony and cartilaginous dorsum. Otolaryngol Clin North Am 1975;8:575–98.

7. Koppe T, Giotakis EI, Heppt W. Functional anatomy of the nose. Facial Plast Surg 2011;27:135–45.

8. Lang J. Clinical anatomy of the nose, nasal cavity, and paranasal sinuses. Stuttgart (Germany): Thieme; 1989.

9. McKinney P, Johnson P, Walloch J. Anatomy of the nasal hump. Plast Reconstr Surg 1986;77:404–5.

10. Bloom JD, Antunes MB, Becker DG. Anatomy, physiology, and general concepts in nasal reconstruction. Facial Plast Surg Clin North Am 2011;19:1–11.

11. Griesman B. Muscles and cartilage of the nose from the standpoint of typical rhinoplasty. Arch Otolaryngol Head Neck Surg 1944;39:334.

12. Williams PL, Warwick R, Dysen M, et al. Gray's anatomy. Edinburgh (United Kingdom): Churchill Livingstone; 1989.

13. Dion MC, Jafek BW, Tobin CE. The anatomy of the nose. External support. Arch Otolaryngol 1978;104:145–50.

14. Gunter JP. Anatomical observations of the lower lateral cartilages. Arch Otolaryngol 1969;89:599–601.

15. Anderson JR. The dynamics of rhinoplasty proceedings of the Ninth International Congress of Otolaryngology. Amsterdam (The Netherlands): Excerpta Medica; 1969.

16. Westreich RW, Lawson W. The tripod theory of nasal tip support revisited: the cantilevered spring model. Arch Facial Plast Surg 2008;10:170–9.

17. Westreich R, Burstein D, Fraser M. The effect of facial asymmetry on nasal deviation. In: Sclafani A, editor. Rhinoplsty: the experts' reference. New York: Thieme; 2015. p. 12–23.

18. Khosh MM, Jen A, Honrado C, et al. Nasal valve reconstruction: experience in 53 consecutive patients. Arch Facial Plast Surg 2004;6:167–71.

19. Park SS, Becker SS. Repair of nasal obstruction in revision rhinoplasty. In: Becker DG, Park SS, editors. Revision rhinoplasty. New York: Thieme; 2008. p. 52–68.

20. Constantian MB. The incompetent external nasal valve: pathophysiology and treatment in primary and secondary rhinoplasty. Plast Reconstr Surg 1994;93:919–31 [discussion: 932–3].

21. Friedman O, Koch CA, Smith WR. Functional support of the nasal tip. Facial Plast Surg 2012;28:225–30.

22. Gassner HG, Sherris DA, Friedman O. Rhinology in rhinoplasty. In: Papel I, editor. Facial plastic and reconstructive surgery. New York: Thieme; 2009. p. 489–506.

23. Schlosser RJ, Park SS. Surgery for the dysfunctional nasal valve. Cadaveric analysis and clinical outcomes. Arch Facial Plast Surg 1999;1:105–10.

24. Cole P. The four components of the nasal valve. Am J Rhinol 2003;17:107–10.

25. Sheen JH. Spreader graft: a method of reconstructing the roof of the middle nasal vault following rhinoplasty. Plast Reconstr Surg 1984;73:230–9.

26. Gray H. The inferior nasal concha. In: Lewis W, editor. Anatomy of the human body. Phildelphia: Lea & Febiger; 2000. Available at: www.bartleby.com/107/.

27. Lam SM, Williams EF 3rd. Anatomic considerations in aesthetic rhinoplasty. Facial Plast Surg 2002;18:209–14.

28. Teller DC. Anatomy of a rhinoplasty: emphasis on the middle third of the nose. Facial Plast Surg 1997;13:241–52.

29. Oneal RM, Beil RJ. Surgical anatomy of the nose. Clin Plast Surg 2010;37:191–211.

30. Mitz V, Peyronie M. The superficial musculoaponeurotic system (SMAS) in the parotid and cheek area. Plast Reconstr Surg 1976;58:80–8.

31. Saban Y, Andretto Amodeo C, Hammou JC, et al. An anatomical study of the nasal superficial musculoaponeurotic system: surgical applications in rhinoplasty. Arch Facial Plast Surg 2008;10:109–15.

32. Toriumi DM, Mueller RA, Grosch T, et al. Vascular anatomy of the nose and the external rhinoplasty approach. Arch Otolaryngol Head Neck Surg 1996;122:24–34.

33. Boahene K, Orten S, Hilger P. Facial analysis of the rhinoplasty patient. In: Papel I, editor. Facial plastic and reconstructive surgery. New York: Thieme; 2009. p. 477–88.

34. Larrabee WF Jr. Facial analysis for rhinoplasty. Otolaryngol Clin North Am 1987;20:653–74.

35. Woodard CR, Park SS. Nasal and facial analysis. Clin Plast Surg 2010;37:181–9.

36. Burres S. Tip points: defining the tip. Aesthetic Plast Surg 1999;23:113–8.

37. Crumley RL, Lanser M. Quantitative analysis of nasal tip projection. Laryngoscope 1988;98:202–8.

38. Milgrim LM, Lawson W, Cohen AF. Anthropometric analysis of the female Latino nose. Revised aesthetic concepts and their surgical implications. Arch Otolaryngol Head Neck Surg 1996;122:1079–86.

39. Ofodile FA, Bokhari FJ, Ellis C. The black American nose. Ann Plast Surg 1993;31:209–18 [discussion: 218–9].

40. Porter JP, Olson KL. Anthropometric facial analysis of the African American woman. Arch Facial Plast Surg 2001;3:191–7.

41. Sim RS, Smith JD, Chan AS. Comparison of the aesthetic facial proportions of southern Chinese

and white women. Arch Facial Plast Surg 2000;2: 113–20.

42. Palma P, Khodaei I, Tasman A. A guide to the assessment and analysis of the rhinoplasty patient. In: Sclafani A, editor. Rhinoplasty: the experts' reference. New York: Thieme; 2015. p. 27–37.

43. Stewart MG, Witsell DL, Smith TL, et al. Development and validation of the Nasal Obstruction Symptom Evaluation (NOSE) scale. Otolaryngol Head Neck Surg 2004;130:157–63.

44. Lipan MJ, Most SP. Development of a severity classification system for subjective nasal obstruction. JAMA Facial Plast Surg 2013;15:358–61.

45. Rhee JS, Sullivan CD, Frank DO, et al. A systematic review of patient-reported nasal obstruction scores: defining normative and symptomatic ranges in surgical patients. JAMA Facial Plast Surg 2014;16: 219–25 [quiz: 232].

46. Stewart MG, Smith TL, Weaver EM, et al. Outcomes after nasal septoplasty: results from the Nasal Obstruction Septoplasty Effectiveness (NOSE) study. Otolaryngol Head Neck Surg 2004;130:283–90.

47. Rhee JS, Poetker DM, Smith TL, et al. Nasal valve surgery improves disease-specific quality of life. Laryngoscope 2005;115:437–40.

48. Most SP. Analysis of outcomes after functional rhinoplasty using a disease-specific quality-of-life instrument. Arch Facial Plast Surg 2006;8:306–9.

49. Palesy T, Pratt E, Mrad N, et al. Airflow and patient-perceived improvement following rhinoplastic correction of external nasal valve dysfunction. JAMA Facial Plast Surg 2015;17:131–6.

50. Kahveci OK, Miman MC, Yucel A, et al. The efficiency of Nose Obstruction Symptom Evaluation (NOSE) scale on patients with nasal septal deviation. Auris Nasus Larynx 2012;39:275–9.

51. Thomas AJ, Orlandi RR, Ashby S, et al. Nasal obstruction has a limited impact on sleep quality and quality of life in patients with chronic rhinosinusitis. Laryngoscope 2016;126(9):1971–6.

52. Hsu HC, Tan CD, Chang CW, et al. Evaluation of nasal patency by visual analogue scale/nasal obstruction symptom evaluation questionnaires and anterior active rhinomanometry after septoplasty: a retrospective one-year follow-up cohort study. Clin Otolaryngol 2017;42(1):53–9.

53. Rhee JS, Arganbright JM, McMullin BT, et al. Evidence supporting functional rhinoplasty or nasal valve repair: A 25-year systematic review. Otolaryngol Head Neck Surg 2008;139:10–20.

54. Kim DW, Rodriguez-Bruno K. Functional rhinoplasty. Facial Plast Surg Clin North Am 2009;17: 115–31, vii.

55. Spielmann PM, White PS, Hussain SS. Surgical techniques for the treatment of nasal valve collapse: a systematic review. Laryngoscope 2009;119:1281–90.

56. Fung E, Hong P, Moore C, et al. The effectiveness of modified cottle maneuver in predicting outcomes in functional rhinoplasty. Plast Surg Int 2014;2014: 618313.

57. Ishii LE, Rhee JS. Are diagnostic tests useful for nasal valve compromise? Laryngoscope 2013;123:7–8.

58. Wittkopf M, Wittkopf J, Ries WR. The diagnosis and treatment of nasal valve collapse. Curr Opin Otolaryngol Head Neck Surg 2008;16:10–3.

59. Strub B, Meuli-Simmen C, Bessler S. Photodocumentation in rhinoplasty surgery. Eur J Plast Surg 2013;36:141–8.

60. Sanchez H, Nuno C, Sanudo E, et al. Correlation between rhinomanometry and NOSE scale measurement of therapeutic success in nasal obstruction. Otolaryngol Head Neck Surg 2014; 151:P115–6.

61. Hilberg O, Jackson AC, Swift DL, et al. Acoustic rhinometry: evaluation of nasal cavity geometry by acoustic reflection. J Appl Physiol (1985) 1989;66:295–303.

62. Lee MK, Most SP. Evidence-Based Medicine: Rhinoplasty. Facial Plast Surg Clin North Am 2015;23: 303–12.

63. Cannon DE, Rhee JS. Evidence-based practice: functional rhinoplasty. Otolaryngol Clin North Am 2012;45:1033–43.

64. Poetker DM, Rhee JS, Mocan BO, et al. Computed tomography technique for evaluation of the nasal valve. Arch Facial Plast Surg 2004;6:240–3.

65. Bloom JD, Sridharan S, Hagiwara M, et al. Reformatted computed tomography to assess the internal nasal valve and association with physical examination. Arch Facial Plast Surg 2012;14:331–5.

66. Lee DC, Shin JH, Kim SW, et al. Anatomical analysis of nasal obstruction: nasal cavity of patients complaining of stuffy nose. Laryngoscope 2013;123:1381–4.

67. Frank-Ito DO, Kimbell JS, Laud P, et al. Predicting postsurgery nasal physiology with computational modeling: current challenges and limitations. Otolaryngol Head Neck Surg 2014;151:751–9.

68. Kimbell JS, Garcia GJ, Frank DO, et al. Computed nasal resistance compared with patient-reported symptoms in surgically treated nasal airway passages: a preliminary report. Am J Rhinol Allergy 2012;26:e94–8.

69. Wang de Y, Lee HP, Gordon BR. Impacts of fluid dynamics simulation in study of nasal airflow physiology and pathophysiology in realistic human three-dimensional nose models. Clin Exp Otorhinolaryngol 2012;5:181–7.

70. Gassner HG, Remington WJ, Sherris DA. Quantitative study of nasal tip support and the effect of reconstructive rhinoplasty. Arch Facial Plast Surg 2001;3:178–84.

71. Beaty MM, Dyer WK 2nd, Shawl MW. The quantification of surgical changes in nasal tip support. Arch Facial Plast Surg 2002;4:82–91.

Septoplasty
Basic and Advanced Techniques

Sam P. Most, MD[a], Shannon F. Rudy, MD[b],*

KEYWORDS

- Nasal septum • Nasal obstruction • Septoplasty • Extracorporeal septoplasty
- Anterior septal reconstruction

KEY POINTS

- Nasal septoplasty is one of the most common procedures in otolaryngology owing to the high prevalence of nasal obstruction from septal deviation.
- Traditional septoplasty is often inadequate in addressing nasal obstruction owing to anterior septal deviation, even when performed in conjunction with techniques to address nasal valve stenosis.
- Extracorporeal resection allows for correction of severe anterocaudal septal deviation but carries a risk of notching at the rhinion.
- Anterior septal reconstruction is a modified extracorporeal septoplasty technique that has been shown to address anterior septal deviation and minimize dorsal deformity and internal nasal valve collapse.

INTRODUCTION

Septal deviation is one of the most common causes of nasal obstruction and a prevalent problem among the general population.[1] As such, septoplasty is among the most frequently performed procedures in otolaryngology and facial plastic surgery. This article provides a brief review of indications for septoplasty, surgical anatomy, and operative technique. We discuss basic and more advanced methods, with a special emphasis on advanced techniques, such as anterior septal reconstruction (ASR) for repair of anterior septal deviation.

SEPTAL ANATOMY

A thorough understanding of the anatomy and function of the nasal septum and its surrounding structures is critical for surgical success. The nasal septum sits in the sagittal plane, extending from the maxillary crest inferiorly to the skull base superiorly and from the nasal tip anteriorly to the nasopharynx posteriorly and divides the nose into 2 nasal cavities.

The nasal septum is composed of both bony and cartilaginous components. Bony components include the maxillary crest, whose anterior extent forms the nasal spine, the perpendicular plate of the ethmoid bone, and the vomer (**Fig. 1**). The quadrangular cartilage (QC) comprises the cartilaginous component and extends to the caudal-most aspect of the septum. Important landmarks of the QC include the anterior and posterior septal angles. Note that the former may extend beyond the nasal spine (see **Fig. 1**). The lateral aspects of the septal bones and cartilage are covered in mucoperiosteum and mucoperichondrium, respectively. At the junction of the bony and cartilaginous components lie decussating fibers, which are important to recognize and divide during surgery in maintain

[a] Division of Facial Plastic and Reconstructive Surgery, Department of Otolaryngology–Head and Neck Surgery, Stanford University School of Medicine, 801 Welch Road, Palo Alto, CA 94305, USA; [b] Department of Otolaryngology—Head and Neck Surgery, Stanford University School of Medicine, 801 Welch Road, Palo Alto, CA 94305, USA
* Corresponding author.
E-mail address: flynns@stanford.edu

facialplastic.theclinics.com

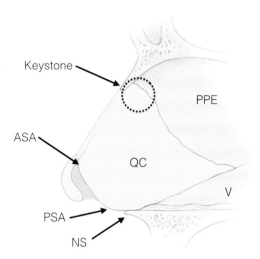

Fig. 1. Basic septal anatomy. The septum itself is composed of the quadrangular cartilage (QC), the perpendicular plate of the ethmoid (PPE), and the vomer (V). The keystone is the major support mechanism of the L-strut, and must be maintained for dorsal and tip support. The anterior and posterior septal angle (ASA and PSA, respectively) and nasal spine (NS) are all important landmarks in septoplasty.

the appropriate subperiosteal and subperichondrial plane and prevent flap perforation.

The "keystone area" is the term that has been given to the attachment of the QC to the bony septum and nasal bones at the rhinion (see **Fig. 1**).[2] Destabilization of this area can result in compromised dorsal integrity with saddle nose deformity.[3] This complication is discussed in more detail below as one of the challenges of reconstruction of the severely deviated septum.

Important Surrounding Structures

Important surrounding structures that must be assessed and, if necessary, addressed during septoplasty include several bony and soft tissue structures. Perhaps the most important of these are the paired upper lateral cartilages, which attach to the cartilaginous septum dorsally. The angle between these and the septum forms the internal nasal valve usually measuring between 10° and 15°. This region is the most narrow point of the anterior nasal airway and is thus of high functional significance with regard to nasal obstruction. High septal deviations can result in narrowing of the internal valve.

The paired lower cartilages, whose medial crural attachments to the septum are 1 of 3 major tip support mechanisms. Note that release of the mucoperichondrium around the anterocaudal

septum necessarily releases this attachment and deprojects the tip. Finally, the inferior turbinates are paired structures that help to regulate nasal airflow. When hypertrophied, they can contribute to nasal obstruction and are often reduced at the time of septoplasty. These structures are reviewed elsewhere in this volume and are not discussed further in this article.

PREOPERATIVE CONSIDERATIONS
Surgical Indications

The most common indication for septoplasty is septal deviation with correlated symptomatic nasal obstruction. Note that a deviated septum alone (ie, without symptomatic obstruction) is not an indication for septoplasty. Other indications include improved access for endoscopic sinus surgery, lead point headaches, and source of graft (cartilage, bone, or mucosal) for patients undergoing skull base surgery.[4]

Preoperative Workup

A thorough preoperative workup is essential for maximizing the potential for benefit and minimizing the risk of complication. Pertinent components of the patient interview include an analysis of symptomatic severity. In our practice, we routinely administer the Nasal Obstructive Symptom Evaluation (NOSE) or Rhinoplasty Health Inventory and Nasal Outcomes scale questionnaire.[5,6] Patients with scaled NOSE scores of less than 30 are classified as "mild" obstruction and are unlikely to be operative candidates.[7] A history of maxillofacial trauma or previous nasal surgery, autoimmune disease, drug use, bleeding disorders, use of anticoagulants, or systemic steroids is noted. Use of intranasal steroids is usually required by most insurance companies before surgical authorization in the United States at this time, and thus we recommend clearly documenting type of intransal steroid use, when used, and duration of use in the history.[8]

Finally, it is of utmost importance that the surgeon determine if the patient currently or previously used vasoconstrictive nasal sprays or illicit drugs intranasally. There is some evidence to suggest that the use of these drugs can increase the risk of septal perforation.[9] The senior author recommends discontinuance of the former for 6 months, and the latter for 1 year before surgery. Moreover, for the latter, we typically ask for a drug screen at the time of preoperative evaluation. Our experience is that patients are very eager to comply with these requests. Photodocumentation of nasal form with standard rhinoplasty views is recommended, although not required of septoplasty patients.[10] If patients desire concomitant aesthetic surgery of the nose, a full rhinoplasty consultation ensues.

Preoperative Physical Examination

In addition to a full head and neck examination, anterior rhinoscopy with a nasal speculum is performed to visualize the nasal septum, as well as the nasal valves. Flexible or rigid nasal endoscopy can complement anterior rhinoscopy but, in this author's experience, is not usually necessary. Mucosal status, as well as the size, of the turbinates are noted. Some key findings to note on examination are: (1) the location, degree, and direction of septal deviation (ie, parallel or perpendicular to plane of the septum), (2) Any posterior nasal spurs, which occur with abnormal bony growth under the posterior QC extension,[11] (3) presence of septal perforation, (4) degree of inferior turbinate hypertrophy, (5) presence or absence of internal nasal valve stenosis (assessed with the modified Cottle maneuver), (6) any internal valve narrowing or lateral wall insufficiency which, if present is noted and graded,[12] (7) the degree of tip support, and (8) any external deformities of the nose, especially dorsal and caudal deviations.

SURGICAL TECHNIQUE

Septoplasty can be performed either with a headlight and nasal speculum, or endoscopically. There are advantages and disadvantages to both techniques, but both have been shown to be successful means by which to correct septal deviation.[13] Regardless of which approach is selected, the same basic surgical technique applies for traditional septoplasty, that is, that involving mild to moderate deviation of the mid or posterior septum.

Standard Endonasal Septoplasty Procedure Outlined

- The patient's nose is first decongested with oxymetazoline in the preoperative holding area. After anesthesia is induced, 1% lidocaine with epinephrine is injected into the mucosa. In addition to providing local anesthetic and vasoconstriction, this injection, when done properly, can result in hydrodissection of the mucoperichondrium off of the septal cartilage, which facilitates flap elevation.
- Next, using a nasal speculum for exposure, a 15-blade scalpel is used to incise the mucosa at the caudal septum down to the level of the cartilage. Either a Killian or hemitransfixion incision can be used; a hemitransfixion incision is more caudally positioned than a Killian

incision and is preferred when caudal deviation is present (**Fig. 2**).

- After making the incision, the senior author typically cross-hatches and scrapes the caudal QC to ensure the proper plane for flap development. After this, a sharp, curved elevator, such as a Cottle elevator, is used to elevate a mucoperichondrial flap. As this flap is raised broadly in the anterior to posterior direction, a blunt elevator such as a Freer elevator may be used. Note that, for standard septoplasty, dissection around the anterocaudal septum is usually not required. However, for caudal deviations, transition around the posterior septal angle is performed and the same plane dissected on the opposite side. If no external approach is planned, restoration of tip support with a septocolumellar stitch is required.
- Next, the surgeon must visualize and mark, if necessary, a 10- to 15-mm strut of cartilage dorsally and caudally. Two important issues must be mentioned. First, it is wise to preserve more than 10 mm (the senior authors prefers 15) at the keystone. In fact, if the septal deviation being treated is located inferiorly, the dorsal incision line of the septum is made must above it, preserving as much nondeviated septal cartilage as possible. Second, the posterior septal angle may exist anterior

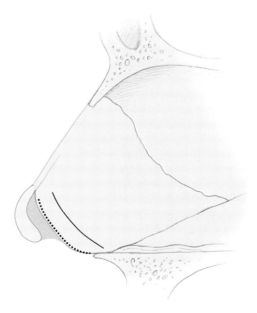

Fig. 2. Incisions used in septoplasty. The hemitransfixion is more caudally positioned (*dotted line*) compared with the Killian incision (*solid line*).

to the nasal spine (see **Fig. 1**), and the caudal strut must include 10 mm over the nasal spine. Thus, the caudal strut may be wider than 10 mm. Once the incision line is marked or visualized clearly, the QC is incised parallel to the dorsum from the keystone anteriorly and then angled inferiorly to define the new L-strut.

- A contralateral mucoperichondrial flap is then raised through this incision again first with a Cottle and then with a Freer elevator. After the bilateral flaps have been elevated, a determination is made regarding bony deviations (these are typically continuous with any QC deviations). The bony septum is incised carefully with a through-biting instrument with care taken not to (1) torque on the skull base or (2) release the keystone.
- The incised cartilage and bone is then removed en bloc using a noncutting instrument such as a Takahashi or bayonet forceps. Any remaining bony spurs can then be removed using a through-biting instrument, with care taken again to avoid torqueing the skull base or keystone support.
- Once all areas of septal deviation have been addressed adequately, the elevated flaps are laid back down. Care must be taken to assess for mucosal perforations and to ensure that, if present, these are not overlapping because this can result in permanent septal perforation. The senior author usually closes any

linear perforations with fine chromic sutures. If opposing tears occurred, both sides are closed meticulously, and intervening tissue (such as morselized septal cartilage) is replaced between the flaps.

- Finally, the mucosal flaps are reapproximated and the mucosal incision is then closed. Surgeon preference dictates if, and what type, of packing or splinting is placed. The senior author performs a quilting suture and uses silastic splints in most septoplasty patients.

ANTERIOR SEPTAL DEVIATION

In cases of mild to moderate mid or posterior septal deviation, the standard septoplasty approach described provides significant benefit in nasal obstruction for most patients.[14] However, deviation of the severely deviated septum, and specifically deviation of the anterocaudal nasal septum, poses unique anatomic and structural challenges that make repair far more challenging.[15–19] Anterocaudal septal deviation can be the result of congenital, traumatic, or iatrogenic insults. This type of septal deviation can be classified as occurring either perpendicular or parallel to the plane of the QC (**Fig. 3**).

Challenges of Anterocaudal Deviation

There are several challenges inherent to correction of anterocaudal septal deviation. First, this condition tends to result in stenosis of the internal nasal

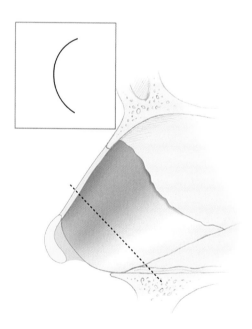 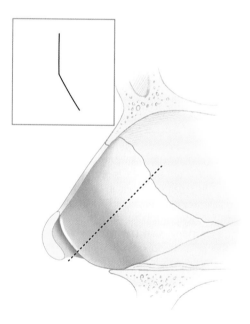

Fig. 3. Anterocaudal septal deviation can occur in a plane that is either perpendicular (*left*) or parallel (*right*) to the quadrangular cartilage. Deviation can also occur simultaneously in both planes.

valves. Second, the location of this type of deviation often results in aesthetic deformity of the nose, including dorsal or columellar irregularities and tip ptosis. Finally, the involvement of the caudal cartilage in anterocaudal septal deviation places nasal tip support mechanisms at risk when repair is attempted.

Repair of anterocaudal septal deviation can be summarized with 2 major goals. First, the nasal airway must be improved through reduction of the deviation. Second, repair must be done in a way such that nasal tip support is not jeopardized.

Management Strategies in Anterocadual Deviation

In light of these myriad factors, traditional septoplasty methods, such as that outlined, often prove inadequate. In response, several more advanced treatment strategies have been described to address anterocaudal septal deviation successfully. Perhaps the best known and studied is the extracorporeal resection, which was first described by King and Ashely in 1952, and is discussed in more detail elsewhere in this article.[20] Preceding this method, Metzenbaum[21] first addressed correction of the caudal septum in 1929 with his description of the "swinging door technique" in which a vertical piece of cartilage is removed from the deviated side with subsequent repositioning of the caudal septum toward midline. Another method that has been described is the translocation technique in which the deviated caudal septum is accessed via a hemitransfixion incision, repositioned to midline, and positioned with polydioxanone sutures.[22] In this technique, no cartilage is removed and thus the septum is not weakened.

Other means by which to repair anterocaudal septal deviation include scoring incisions, spreader grafts, morselization of septal cartilage, tongue-in-groove stabilization, batten grafts, the use of biosynthetic material such as polydioxanone foil as a matrix for reconstruction in conjunction with pieces of native septal cartilage, use of costal and/or conchal cartilage grafts, and use of nonautologus materials such as Medipore and silicone.[23]

Although all of these techniques have been shown to have varying degrees of benefit in the correctly identified patient, repositioning and suturing methods such as those described are often inadequate in addressing severe caudal septal deviation and associated internal nasal valve stenosis, which thus require more involved reconstruction techniques. One reason for this is that, if the septum is fundamentally misshapen, even

repositioning the caudal aspect to the midline will inadequately treat either the nasal obstruction, aesthetic concerns, or both.

EXTRACORPOREAL RESECTION

As its name implies, the guiding principal of extracorporeal resection is removal of the entire nasal septum to correct severe deviation. Although this has been described as an endoscopic procedure, today this is typically addressed via an external rhinoplasty approach. The procedure has been extensively described by Gubisch.[24] As detailed by Gubisch, this procedure can be described in 3 distinct stages, the first of which is exposure and removal of the native septum. The first stage begins with a hemitransfixion incision that is extended to an intracartilaginous incision to provide optimal exposure. After the anterior border of the septum is exposed, dissection is then carried out along the more concave side of the septum. The border of the septum with the upper lateral cartilages is then exposed and the septum is freed from this junction. The mucoperichondrium is then freed from the more convex side of the septum. The anterior nasal spine is then exposed and the septum is freed from the premaxilla below and removed en bloc. The second stage involves nasal tip and bony pyramid correction, as well as reconstruction of the removed septum in creating as straight as possible a septum, which is accomplished through the use of interrupted sutures, release of intracartilaginous tension lines, and rasping. The final stage involves reimplantation of the septum and recreation of an ideal nasolabial angle using the tongue and groove technique between the septum and nasal spine. Once ideal positioning has been achieved, the implant is secured in place with transseptal sutures.

Although Gubisch has shown excellent results with this technique, a revision rate of 9% is noted, and has been mitigated by routine inclusion of camouflage grafts to mask settling at the rhinion. The reason for this is the technical challenge in reforming the bony–cartilaginous attachment at the keystone that forms the familiar dorsal line on profile. Any minute irregularity here is visible to the naked eye.

ANTERIOR SEPTAL RECONSTRUCTION

In light of the aesthetic deformity and difficulty with keystone reconstruction associated with extracorporeal resection, Most[25] has described a modified form of extracorporeal resection, called ASR. ASR follows the same general principles as standard extracorporeal resection with the key distinction that in ASR, a dorsal strut is preserved (**Fig. 4**). This allows for the ability to correct severe and anterocaudal septal deviation, unlike with standard septoplasty, while minimizing the risks of nasal collapse and notching at the rhinion that are associated with extracorporeal resection.

Anterior Septal Reconstruction Technique

- The procedure is begun with a left-sided hemitransfixion incision regardless of the laterality of septal deviation. Bilateral submucoperichondrial flaps are then elevated around the anterior septum as described in the standard septoplasty technique.
- Once this exposure is completed, the degree of deviation is assessed to confirm the preoperative determination that traditional septoplasty will be inadequate. After this confirmation, conversion to open rhinoplasty is undertaken.
- Next, the upper lateral cartilages are exposed and released from the septum, which is viewed from above.
- A significant portion of the QC is then resected (**Fig. 5**). However, unlike the traditional extracorporeal resection, a dorsal strut is maintained, which is variable in length, but measures at least 2 cm. The strut is designed to have a height of 1.5 cm in the vertical direction at the keystone area, tapering to 1 cm anteriorly.
- The attachment of the septum to the nasal bones at the keystone area is critical in providing support for the subsequent ASR

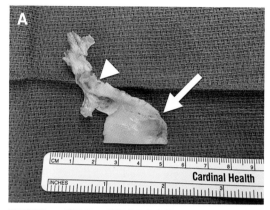

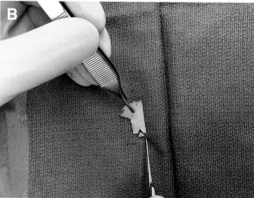

Fig. 5. Intraoperative images for anterior septal reconstruction. (*A*) Subtotal resection of septum. Arrowhead, posterior quadrangular cartilage extension. Arrow, posterior septal angle. (*B*) A notch is created in the anterior septal reconstruction graft to fit into the maxillary spine.

graft and for maintaining a natural dorsal profile and must be preserved.
- If bony deviation is present, this is removed in continuity with the cartilaginous septum.
- The resected cartilage is then analyzed and constructed into the graft, using the straightest portion when possible
- Should the resected cartilage prove insufficient for grafting, an autologous rib graft is obtained. As of this writing, the senior author routinely offers autologous rib graft to all patients. For patients over 60 years of age, this is done with the understanding that if no noncalcified costal cartilage if found at surgery, homologous irradiated rib grafts may be required.
- The posterior septal angle is then fixed. This is accomplished by exposing the anterior nasal spine with monopolar cautery, with care to preserve the overlying periosteum, and then using a 2- to 4-mm osteotome to split the

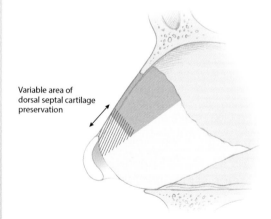

Variable area of dorsal septal cartilage preservation

Fig. 4. The cartilage delineated in purple represents the strut that is always preserved. The stippled area represents cartilage that is variably resected.

spine to a depth of 2 to 3 mm (**Fig. 6**). In some cases, the spine may already have a groove and thus no osteotomy is required.

- A notch is created posterior to the posterior septal angle of the ASR graft and this notch is placed subsequently into the groove created in the nasal spine (**Fig. 7**) on the concave side of the midvault. The notching technique prevents both anteroposterior and lateral displacement of the graft, and is confirmed by the surgeon. If this is not secured, an absorbable polydioxanone suture is placed through the neoposterior septal angle and the preserved periosteum.
- To secure the ASR graft to the preserved dorsal strut, 5-0 nonabsorbable monofilament sutures are used and tongue-in-groove stabilization is performed between the medial crura and the ASR using a 5-0 nonabsorbable monofilament suture (see **Fig. 7**). Rarely, a single 5-0 absorbable monofilament suture is used to secure the graft to the overlying periosteum of the spine.
- To repair the upper lateral cartilages to the dorsum, a 5-0 nonabsorbable monofilament suture is then used. The tip is repaired with dome-binding sutures. If additional tip support is indicated, an alar spanning suture is placed. The external rhinoplasty incision is

closed with 6-0 nonabsorbable suture externally and 5-0 chromic suture intransally.

- The hemistransfixion incision is closed, and quilting sutures placed, as in a standard septoplasty. Intranasal silastic splints are placed and secured to the ASR graft using a through-and-through 4-0 nonabsorbable monofilament suture. The nose is taped and a thermoplastic splint placed. The intranasal silastic splints, columellar sutures, external tape, and splint are removed 1 week postoperatively.

PATIENT OUTCOMES IN ANTERIOR SEPTAL RECONSTRUCTION

In the senior author's original description of 12 patients, nasal obstructive symptoms were reduced significantly as measured by NOSE scores. Subsequently, Surowitz and colleagues[26] analyzed 77 patients who underwent ASR. Septal cartilage was used for the ASR graft in 60 cases, autologous rib in 7 cases, and homologous irradiated rib in 10 cases. There was a statistically significant difference between NOSE scores, both between the preoperative mean (68.2) and early postoperative mean (21.1) scores, as well as between the preoperative mean and late postoperative mean (15.8) NOSE scores in patients who underwent ASR. In

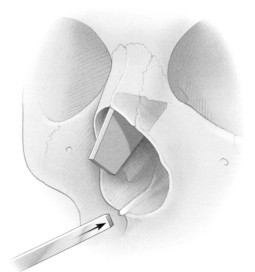
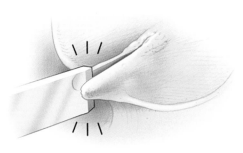

Osteotome is used to gently divide the anterior portion of the maxillary spine

Fig. 6. Creation of the maxillary spine recipient site. The dorsal septal remnant is shown in purple (*left*). Right, Use of a straight osteotome to split the maxillary spine with gentle or no tapping.

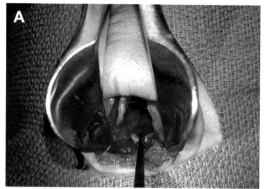

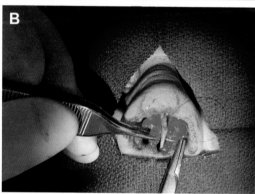

Fig. 7. Intraoperative images for anterior septal reconstruction. (A) A 3-mm straight osteotome is used to divide the anterior-most maxillary spine. (B) Tongue-in-groove reconstruction of tip support to the anterior septal reconstruction graft.

adequate for individuals with mild to moderate mid to posterior septal deviation, unique challenges arise with caudal septal deviation, especially when this is severe. Herein, multiple strategies that attempt to address anterior septal deviation have been discussed. ASR, described by the senior author just over a decade ago, has been shown to be a safe and effective means by which to address severe caudal septal deviation and long-term reduction in preoperative symptoms.

ACKNOWLEDGMENTS

Medical illustrations by Christine Gralapp, MA, CMI.

REFERENCES

1. Fettman N, Sanford T, Sindwani R. Surgical management of the deviated septum: techniques in septoplasty. Otolaryngol Clin North Am 2009;42(2): 241–52, viii.
2. Simon PE, Lam K, Sidle D, et al. The nasal keystone region: an anatomical study. JAMA Facial Plast Surg 2013;15(3):235–7.
3. Gubisch W, Constantinescu MA. Refinements in extracorporal septoplasty. Plast Reconstr Surg 1999; 104(4):1131–9 [discussion: 1140–2].
4. Kennedy DW, Hwang PH. Rhinology: diseases of the nose, sinuses, and skull base. New York: Thieme; 2012.
5. Stewart MG, Witsell DL, Smith TL, et al. Development and validation of the Nasal Obstruction Symptom Evaluation (NOSE) scale. Otolaryngol Head Neck Surg 2004;130(2):157–63.
6. Lee MK, Most SP. A comprehensive quality-of-life instrument for aesthetic and functional rhinoplasty: the RHINO scale. Plast Reconstr Surg Glob open 2016; 4(2):e611.
7. Lipan MJ, Most SP. Development of a severity classification system for subjective nasal obstruction. JAMA Facial Plast Surg 2013;15(5):358–61.
8. Teti VP, Akdagli S, Most SP. Cost-effectiveness of corticosteroid nasal spray vs surgical therapy in patients with severe to extreme anatomical nasal obstruction. JAMA Facial Plast Surg 2016;18(3):165–70.
9. Cervin A, Andersson M. Intranasal steroids and septum perforation–an overlooked complication? A description of the course of events and a discussion of the causes. Rhinology 1998;36(3):128–32.
10. Swamy RS, Most SP. Pre- and postoperative portrait photography: standardized photos for various procedures. Facial Plast Surg Clin North Am 2010; 18(2):245–52. Table of Contents.
11. Saedi B, Rashan AR, Lipan M, et al. Consistent ipsilateral development of the posterior extension of the quadrangular cartilage and bony spur formation in

this series, 3 postoperative complications were identified: warping of an autologous rib graft in 1 patient, palate hypoesthesia at 7 months in 1 patient, and nasal tip hypoesthesia at 1 year in 1 patient.

Importantly, the studies by Surowitz and colleagues[26] and Teti and colleagues[8] have demonstrated no discernable benefit from requiring patients with documented severe septal deviation to use intranasal steroids before authorization for surgery. It is the senior author's hope that such studies will allow better health care delivery by eliminating unnecessary medication use and physician visits for such patients.

SUMMARY

Nasal septal deviation is a prevalent problem that can have significant quality of life ramifications in affected individuals. Septoplasty is a commonly performed procedure that provides qualitative and quantitative benefit to many individuals who suffer from nasal obstruction owing to septal deviation. Although a standard, basic technique is often nasal septal deviation. Otolaryngol Head Neck Surg 2015;152(3):444–8.

12. Tsao GJ, Fijalkowski N, Most SP. Validation of a grading system for lateral nasal wall insufficiency. Allergy Rhinol (Providence) 2013;4(2):e66–8.

13. Prepageran N, Lingham OR. Endoscopic septoplasty: the open book method. Indian J Otolaryngol Head Neck Surg 2010;62(3):310–2.

14. Paradis J, Rotenberg BW. Open versus endoscopic septoplasty: a single-blinded, randomized, controlled trial. J Otolaryngol Head Neck Surg 2011;40(Suppl 1): S28–33.

15. Most SP. Analysis of outcomes after functional rhinoplasty using a disease-specific quality-of-life instrument. Arch Facial Plast Surg 2006;8(5):306–9.

16. Most SP. Trends in functional rhinoplasty. Arch Facial Plast Surg 2008;10(6):410–3.

17. Rohrich RJ, Hollier LH. Use of spreader grafts in the external approach to rhinoplasty. Clin Plast Surg 1996;23(2):255–62.

18. Sheen JH. Spreader graft: a method of reconstructing the roof of the middle nasal vault following rhinoplasty. Plast Reconstr Surg 1984;73(2):230–9.

19. Yoo S, Most SP. Nasal airway preservation using the autospreader technique: analysis of outcomes using a disease-specific quality-of-life instrument. Arch Facial Plast Surg 2011;13(4):231–3.

20. King ED, Ashley FL. The correction of the internally and externally deviated nose. Plastic and Reconstr Surg (1946) 1952;10(2):116–20.

21. Metzenbaum M. Replacement of the lower end of the dislocated septal cartilage versus submucous section of the dislocated end of the septal cartilage. Arch Otolaryngol 1929;9:193–282.

22. Sedwick JD, Lopez AB, Gajewski BJ, et al. Caudal septoplasty for treatment of septal deviation: aesthetic and functional correction of the nasal base. Arch Facial Plast Surg 2005;7(3):158–62.

23. Haack J, Papel ID. Caudal septal deviation. Otolaryngol Clin North Am 2009;42(3):427–36.

24. Gubisch W. The extracorporeal septum plasty: a technique to correct difficult nasal deformities. Plast Reconstr Surg 1995;95(4):672–82.

25. Most SP. Anterior septal reconstruction: outcomes after a modified extracorporeal septoplasty technique. Arch Facial Plast Surg 2006;8(3):202–7.

26. Surowitz J, Lee MK, Most SP. Anterior septal reconstruction for treatment of severe caudal septal deviation: clinical severity and outcomes. Otolaryngol Head Neck Surg 2015;153(1):27–33.

The Inferior Turbinate in Rhinoplasty

Brian W. Downs, MD

KEYWORDS

- Inferior turbinate hypertrophy • Nasal obstruction • Rhinoplasty
- Submucous resection of inferior turbinate • Septoplasty

KEY POINTS

- There is controversy regarding optimum treatment of the hypertrophied inferior turbinate.
- Patients undergoing rhinoplasty will likely need treatment of bony hypertrophy as well as possibly soft tissue hypertrophy.
- Although inferior turbinate hypertrophy is a heterogeneous entity, future studies should standardize outcome measures and compare treatment methods with rigorous clinical trials.

INTRODUCTION

Initially, surgery for the nose addressed only the external component. The efforts of surgeons in India to reconstruct nasal defects thousands of years ago are well documented, and Tagliacozzi illustrated dramatic methods of nasal flap reconstruction. The syphilis epidemic of the 1600s and later the First World War provided numerous patients who needed nasal reconstruction as a result of infection and trauma, respectively. Purely aesthetic rhinoplasty was pioneered by Jacques Joseph, who performed surgery on his first patient in 1898.[1] Concurrently, interest in the internal nose also developed. For example, there are reports of inserting a hot poker in the nose to treat nasal obstruction.[2] Then, in the latter part of the nineteenth century, Jones is reported to have had the first description of turbinate surgery (1895).[3] Several years later, Holmes[4] outlined his experience with more than 1500 cases of turbinate resection.

In the early-mid 1900s, inferior turbinate surgery was marked by a period of controversy. Many surgeons thought that turbinate resection resulted in atrophic rhinitis and ozena. As a result, total inferior turbinate resection fell out of favor. A more conservative procedure emerged featuring preservation of anatomy, suggested first by Spielberg,[5] who advocated for submucous resection in 1924.

Flashing forward to today, we have realized the importance of treating both the internal and the external nose at the same time. In a recent survey from the American Society of Plastic Surgeons, 87% of respondents indicated that they would like to see additional instructional courses on the nasal airway.[6] For the nose, function follows form. Inferior turbinate hypertrophy continues to be a clinical focus when evaluating nasal obstruction, and nasal function should be considered for any patient undergoing rhinoplasty surgery. To the extent that septal abnormality is often present in rhinoplasty patients (functional or cosmetic), the author herein also considers articles that discuss the inferior turbinate and septoplasty—often using septoplasty as a proxy for rhinoplasty—as one considers the role of the inferior turbinate in rhinoplasty surgery. Given that the vast majority of rhinoplasty surgeries are performed on adults, studies areconsidered that look at the inferior turbinate in adults only—even though large pediatric studies have been published.[7]

Department of Otolaryngology, Wake Forest Baptist Health, Medical Center Boulevard, Winston-Salem, NC 27157, USA
E-mail address: bdowns@wakehealth.edu

Facial Plast Surg Clin N Am 25 (2017) 171–177
http://dx.doi.org/10.1016/j.fsc.2016.12.003
1064-7406/17/

ANATOMY AND PHYSIOLOGY OF THE INFERIOR TURBINATE

The inferior turbinate is situated as a composite protrusion extending from the internal aspect of the lateral nasal sidewall. Its anterior aspect forms the inferior border of the nasal valve, which is the flow-limiting segment of the nasal airway. The inferior turbinate (conchal) bone is situated superiorly and angled to some degree both medially and inferiorly toward the airway. It has a rough texture to which soft tissue is tightly adherent. The soft tissue of the turbinate is composed of arterial and venous vascular channels as well as smooth muscle.[8] In this way, the turbinate acts as a dynamic erectile organ. Structurally, the inferior turbinate is often seen "curling" around an ipsilateral septal deviation, adopting a lateralized position at the apex of the spur and then becoming more medial anterior and posterior to it (**Fig. 1**A). A curled configuration may suggest some adaptation in shape to the space allotted or to the airflow pattern in the pathologic airway. Conversely, the inferior turbinate contralateral to a septal deviation often becomes hypertrophied, again suggesting an ultrastructural adaptation to available space (**Fig. 1**B). Indeed, Jun and colleagues[9] found that the hypertrophied turbinate on the concave side of a septal deviation features a change in orientation of the conchal bone relative to the lateral nasal sidewall. Specifically, they found that the angle at which the turbinate protrudes from the lateral nasal sidewall demonstrated a statistically significant increase relative to the other side. In other words, the angle of attachment of the turbinate to the nasal is more obtuse on the more open side. It stands to reason that a space-occupying inferior turbinate that juts

out in the airway more could impair subjective airflow.

The blood supply to the inferior turbinate is composed of anterior and posterior contributions. The anterior ethmoid artery and lateral nasal artery provide anterior blood supply, whereas the sphenopalatine artery provides posterior blood supply.[10–12] One anatomic study emphasized the position of the posterior blood supply and its intimate association with the turbinate bone, finding that 2 primary branches supply blood to the turbinate, and that both remain in bony canals or lie in close approximation to the bone for a significant distance. The anterior and posterior blood supply anastamose along the midportion of the turbinate, forming the inferior turbinate artery.[11] The caliber of the blood vessels along this middle aspect of the turbinate has been noted to increase. Larger vessels in this area may represent an anastomosis phenomenon related to the anterior blood supply or could include contribution from the facial artery.[11,13] This robust inferior turbinate blood supply allows for use of the inferior turbinate flap in various reconstructive procedures.[12,14]

The function of the inferior turbinate is to warm and humidify the air that is breathed. As air passes through the nasal valve, it is directed toward the surface of the inferior turbinate, underscoring the importance of both structures for nasal breathing. Laminar airflow passing over the turbinate creates resistance, which causes nasal mucus production, thereby providing humidification.[8] The normal nose can increase humidity of respired air from zero externally to near 100% at the level of the nasopharynx.[15] Increased humidity in the nasopharynx would explain significant upper airway dryness symptoms typically associated with total turbinectomy.

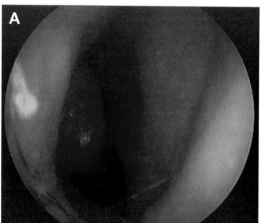 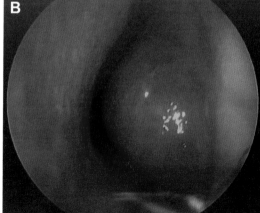

Fig. 1. (*A*) Inferior turbinate position ipsilateral to septal deviation. (*B*) Compensatory inferior turbinate position contralateral to septal deviation.

CAUSES OF INFERIOR TURBINATE HYPERTROPHY

The cause of inferior turbinate enlargement is controversial; many possibilities exist. Indeed, there is even controversy regarding the terminology that should be used when describing this phenomenon. Farmer and Eccles[16] argue that the term "inferior turbinate enlargement" is preferable because there is no true histologic evidence of enlargement of the cells—either bony or soft tissue—which characterizes the definition of hypertrophy. The mucosa is thought by most to play at least a partial role in inferior turbinate hypertrophy. A dynamically enlarged inferior turbinate can result from the engorgement of the vascular soft tissues of the nose as part of the generally accepted nasal congestion-decongestion cycle. A boggy appearance to the inferior turbinate often is a classic finding in patients who have allergic rhinitis. Indeed, Mabry and Marple[17] emphasized the role of allergy and suggested that failure to shrink after decongestant treatment suggested "irreversible hypertrophy." The use of continuous positive airway pressure has also been anecdotally implicated in turbinate hypertrophy.[18]

Bony enlargement has been implicated in at least some cases of inferior turbinate enlargement.[19] Subsequent retrospective reviews of coronal computed tomographic (CT) scans in patients with compensatory hypertrophy of one inferior turbinate contralateral to a septal deviation showed an increase in cross-sectional area of both bony and mucosal elements as compared with controls, suggesting that treatment of the bone is needed for compensatory hypertrophy.[9,20] Persistent inflammation in the nose can also create collagen deposition and glandular hypertrophy, resulting in permanent thickening in the nasal mucoperiosteum.[21] These studies, combined with Jun's work looking at the angle of protrusion of the turbinate, suggest that, in many cases, modifying the turbinate bone in addition to the vascular soft tissues could help relieve nasal obstruction.

DIAGNOSIS OF INFERIOR TURBINATE HYPERTROPHY

Diagnosis of inferior turbinate hypertrophy is done primarily by physical examination. Anterior rhinoscopy can help determine the angle at which the turbinate attaches to the lateral nasal sidewall. It will also provide information regarding the soft tissue bulk of the turbinate. A wax curette can be used to gently palpate the anterior head of the inferior turbinate to assess soft tissue bulk. If this is poorly tolerated, a topical anesthetic can be placed. With anterior rhinoscopy, simultaneous evaluation can be done in quick succession of the septum as well as the nasal valve. Patients who have prior CT imaging of the sinonasal cavity can undergo radiographic assessment of the inferior turbinates, but ordering new imaging would ordinarily not be indicated. For the inferior turbinate partially obscured by a deviated septum or otherwise difficult to assess, especially posteriorly, nasal endoscopy may be warranted.

TREATMENT FOR INFERIOR TURBINATE HYPERTROPHY
Nonsurgical Treatment

Both surgical and nonsurgical treatments exist for inferior turbinate hypertrophy. Assuming that inferior turbinate hypertrophy can involve not only a soft tissue but also a bony component, it would stand to reason that nonsurgical therapy would be limited to possible improvements in the soft tissue component only—the mucosa and submucosal vascularized spaces—because a spray or pill would not be expected to effectively modify or reposition "hard" tissue such as cartilage or bone. Studies outlining nonsurgical therapy for inferior turbinate hypertrophy use "nasal obstruction" as a proxy given that isolating the effects of systemic treatment on a single intranasal structure is impossible. Patients enrolled in such studies often carry a diagnosis of allergic rhinitis. Knowledge of nonsurgical therapy for nasal obstruction is important for the rhinoplasty surgeon because optimizing the nasal airway by reducing systemic or diffuse inflammation allows for better evaluation of the fixed structure of the nose. Comprehensive treatment of the nose includes controlling for allergy and other inflammatory causes. In addition, the surgeon may be asked to treat nasal obstruction medically before insurance approval for rhinoplasty. Finally, postoperative nasal obstruction after rhinoplasty may call for adjuvant medical therapy.

Even though second-generation oral antihistamines (OAH) remain popular for nonsurgical treatment of nasal obstruction and are easily accessible over the counter, first-line therapy should include intranasal steroid (INS) spray. Steroids have represented a time-tested anchor of nonsurgical therapy for nasal obstruction. Steroid injections into the inferior turbinate were described more than 30 years ago.[22,23] More recently, INSs were developed, and Benninger and colleagues[24] demonstrated in 2010 that treatment of allergic rhinitis symptoms with INS was superior to OAH, intranasal antihistamine spray (IAH), leukotriene receptor antagonists, and cromolyn. Subsequent studies have suggested that IAH may be equivalent, such as a randomized controlled trial comparing INS and IAH.[25] Even though INSs do not seem to represent the higher level risk that systemic steroids do,[26] the true risk of these topical sprays is not known. As with other proposed interventions, proper informed consent is important. When prescribing INS, an effort should be made to discuss possible side effects, such as adrenal suppression, depressed immune function, glaucoma, epistaxis, septal perforation, nasal irritation, and nasal dryness.

Surgical Treatment

A helpful concept to keep in mind when evaluating surgical treatment of the inferior turbinate is whether that treatment is addressing soft tissue, bone, or both. A slender turbinate with an obtuse angle of attachment or thicker bone may require bony work, whereas a boggy turbinate with thickened mucosa and an acute angle of attachment may call primarily for treatment of soft tissue. Certainly, there are combinations of both in which bony and soft tissue abnormality co-exist.

Treating the bone: inferior turbinate lateralization

Modern-day modification of the inferior turbinate bone can include repositioning only (lateralization) or partial removal. Lateralization has been examined in several studies that were summarized nicely by Moss and colleagues[27] in a letter to Plastic and Reconstructive Surgery in 2015. The appeal of lateralization is that it is conservative and anatomy sparing. The perceived downside is that it is not durable.[28] Perhaps the best pure study of turbinate lateralization was done by Aksoy and colleagues.[29] In this study, 40 patients underwent inferior turbinate lateralization only without other turbinate procedures. Thirty-two of these patients also had septoplasty. Preoperative, 1-month, and 6-month radiographic studies were done by CT scan. Findings were remarkable for a statistically significant decrease in the angle of turbinate relative to the lateral nasal sidewall, the distance of the turbinate from the lateral nasal sidewall, and the cross-sectional area lateral to the turbinate. The authors of this study also placed Doyle splints for a week, which could possibly minimize early turbinate remedialization. Admittedly, their follow-up period was short.

Passali and colleagues[30] showed the benefits of lateralization with a fairly large prospective randomized trial. In their study, comparison was made between submucosal resection with and without lateralization, turbinectomy, laser cautery, electrocautery, and cryotherapy. Submucosal resection provided the best results and was statistically significantly better as measured by patient's symptom scores. Adding lateralization to submucosal resection improved symptom scores but did not reach statistical significance. Preservation of nasal physiology, as measured by secretory immunoglobulin A and mucociliary clearance time, was maintained. Notably, 92 of the original 382 patients were included in the 6-year follow-up, providing a relatively robust study group. Similarly, microdebrider-assisted turbinate reduction has been found to deliver favorable outcomes when combined with turbinate outfracture.[31]

Treating the bone: submucosal resection of conchal bone

One of the largest reported series of true submucosal resection of the turbinates has been reported by Rohrich and colleagues.[32] They described fracturing the turbinate laterally, excising a small amount of mucosa inferolaterally, and removing bone along the inferior half of the conchal bone. Their technique seems to be an effective way to reduce the vertical length of the turbinate and open up the inferior nasal airway. Of 281 patients in their study who underwent this procedure, only one had mucosal crusting and none had bleeding, recurrent obstruction, or symptoms of atrophic rhinitis. Even though this procedure reduces the total surface area of inferior turbinate available for warming and humidifying air, the nose generally seems to be able to compensate for a smaller inferior turbinate with minimal symptoms.[33] Durable improvement over a 4-year follow-up has also been reported after submucous resection of conchal bone in allergic rhinitis patients in which all mucosa was preserved and the "mucoperiosteal sack" was cauterized.[34]

Inferior turbinate reduction with concurrent septoplasty

Inferior turbinate hypertrophy frequently coexists with other sinonasal abnormality, including deviated septum, chronic rhinosinusitis, and nasal valve collapse. Performing septoplasty with inferior turbinate reduction is especially common and, based on the aforementioned evidence of enlargement of the contralateral inferior turbinate, it would seem that turbinate reduction would be indicated. Specifically, in a large retrospective review spanning 12 years, there was a statistically significant decrease in the need for revision surgery in patients who underwent simultaneous turbinate reduction at time of primary septoplasty.[35] In contrast, Becker and colleagues[36] showed no benefit of concurrent turbinate reduction at time of primary septoplasty. A recent clinical consensus statement from the American Academy of Otolaryngology–Head and Neck Surgery noted that inferior turbinoplasty is an effective adjunctive procedure to septoplasty, although the tone of the recommendation was guarded.[37]

Inferior turbinectomy

In computer models, total resection of the inferior turbinate increases area within the nose but simultaneously decreases nasal resistance and impairs the ability of the nose to warm and humidify inspired air.[15] Concerns also exist for postoperative bleeding after turbinectomy given the close proximity of arterial blood supply to the bone. Postoperative pain can also occur. Extended follow-up via use of a questionnaire prompted Moore and colleagues[38] to conclude that total turbinectomy should not be performed. However, large retrospective studies suggest relative safety of inferior turbinectomy. Talmon and colleagues[39] reported 357 total inferior turbinectomies performed in a dry climate (Israel) with 6-year follow-up. In this study, there were no cases of atrophic rhinitis, and 348 of 357 reported being "satisfied" with the operation at 6 months. The perioperative bleeding rate was 1.7%, and the 18-month rate of nasal crusting was 3.7%.[39] Moreover, many patients undergoing Le Fort osteotomy have turbinectomy as part of their maxillary repositioning. For example, Movahed and colleagues[40] reported on 603 patients who underwent partial inferior turbinectomy involving two-thirds (presumably anteriorly) of each turbinate. No details are provided, but they emphasized that "chart review showed no significant long-term complications."

Electrosurgery for inferior turbinate enlargement

There is a myriad of studies that examine electrosurgery for inferior turbinate enlargement, and much of this literature is outside the scope of this review. Electrosurgical techniques include cautery (diathermy) of the inferior turbinate, coblation of the inferior turbinate, and radiofrequency ablation of the inferior turbinate.[41–43] Many of these studies examine inferior turbinate enlargement in isolation, often addressed in a clinic setting under local anesthesia, making this body of literature somewhat less relevant for rhinoplasty surgeons who are more likely to proceed to surgery under general anesthesia. Many studies are also weakened by short follow-up periods and lack of standardized outcomes measures.

PROPOSED ALGORITHM FOR TREATMENT OF INFERIOR TURBINATE HYPERTROPHY IN RHINOPLASTY

In general, most patients with inferior turbinate enlargement who are undergoing rhinoplasty will be treated under general anesthesia. The use of general anesthesia allows for a wide range of options and a greater degree of freedom to attenuate not only soft tissue of the turbinate but also the conchal bone. In addition, many rhinoplasty patients present with concurrent septal deviation and associated compensatory (bony?) turbinate enlargement. The literature seems to suggest that the most reasonable treatment is therefore a combination bony/soft tissue surgery. Bony attenuation involves either turbinate outfracture or submucous resection, both of which have a low complication rate, as discussed above. Published studies of total turbinectomy report few complications, but there is contradictory literature to refute this.[44] Treatment of isolated soft tissue enlargement of the turbinate is easily done in an office setting under local anesthesia and may very well fall outside the purview of the rhinoplasty surgeon.

FUTURE DIRECTIONS

Determining the best treatment for inferior turbinate enlargement is complex because of the heterogeneous nature of the disease process, the diverse patient population, and the lack of standardization of equipment used. A recent Cochrane Library publication highlighted the shortcomings of turbinate reduction research studies.[45] Studying turbinate surgery in a population of rhinoplasty patients becomes even more difficult because these patients are, by definition, undergoing other procedures (rhinoplasty, septoplasty) that may contribute to improvement in nasal airway. Lack of agreed-upon outcomes is also an issue, but the NOSE (Nasal Obstruction Symptom Evaluation) scale has been widely used and is generally accepted as one of the best patient self-report instruments.[46]

The inferior turbinate has been found to be a source of human mesenchymal stem cells.[47] As a result, it is possible that some alteration in differentiation of these stem cells could contribute to turbinate hypertrophy and nasal obstruction. Indeed, one study looked at the characterization and differentiation of hypertrophied turbinates versus normal turbinates and found no difference in the mesenchymal stem cells.[48] Future directions in regenerative medicine could search for answers to some of these questions.

REFERENCES

1. Natvig P. Jacques Joseph: surgical sculptor. Philadelphia: W.B. Saunders; 1982.

2. A history of nasal surgery: from the "Indian Nose" to modern septo-rhinoplasty. Boenisch cosmetic surgery. Available at: http://www.nasenchirurgie.at/rhino/medication/nose-surgery/history-of-rhinoplasty/. Accessed July 21, 2016.

3. Jones TC. Turbinotomy. Lancet 1895;2:496.

4. Holmes CR. Hypertrophy of the turbinated bodies. NY Med J 1900;72:529.

5. Spielberg W. The treatment of nasal obstruction by submucosal resection of the inferior turbinate. Laryngoscope 1924;34:197–205.

6. Afifi AM, Kempton SJ, Gordon CR, et al. Evaluating current functional airway surgery during rhinoplasty: a survey of the American Society of Plastic Surgeons. Aesthetic Plast Surg 2015;39:181–90.

7. Arganbright JM, Jensen EL, Mattingly J. Utility of inferior turbinoplasty for the treatment of nasal obstruction in children: a 10-year review. JAMA Otolaryngol Head Neck Surg 2015;141:901–4.

8. King HC, Mabry RL. A practical guide to the management of nasal and sinus disorders. New York: Thieme; 1993.

9. Jun BC, Kim SW, Kim SW. Is turbinate surgery necessary when performing a septoplasty? Eur Arch Otorhinolaryngol 2009;266:975–80.

10. Truex RC, Kellner CE. Detailed atlas of the head and neck. New York: Oxford University Press; 1948.

11. Gil Z, Margalit N. Anteriorly based inferior turbinate flap for endoscopic skull base reconstruction. Otolaryngol Head Neck Surg 2012;146:842–7.

12. Murakami CS, Kriet JD, Ierokomos AP. Nasal reconstruction using the inferior turbinate mucosal flap. Arch Facial Plast Surg 1999;1:97–100.

13. Padgham N, Vaughan-Jones R. Cadaver studies of the anatomy of arterial supply to the inferior turbinates. J R Soc Med 1991;84:728–30.

14. Harvey RJ, Sheahan PO, Schlosser RJ. Inferior turbinate pedicle flap for endoscopic skull base defect repair. Am J Rhinol Allergy 2009;23:522–6.

15. Dayal A, Rhee JS, Garcia GJM. Impact of middle versus inferior total turbinectomy on nasal aerodynamics. Otolaryngol Head Neck Surg 2016;155(3):518–25.

16. Farmer SEJ, Eccles R. Chronic inferior turbinate enlargement and the implications for surgical intervention. Rhinology 2006;44:234–8.

17. Mabry RL, Marple BF. Management of the obstructing inferior turbinate. In: Schaefer SD, editor. Rhinology and sinus disease: a problem oriented approach. St Louis (MO): Mosby; 1998. p. 68.

18. Marks SC. Nasal and sinus surgery. Philadelphia: W.B. Saunders; 2000.

19. Fairbanks DNF, Kaliner M. Nonallergic rhinitis and infection. In: Cummings CW, Fredrickson JM, Harker AL, et al, editors. Otolaryngology head and neck surgery. 3rd edition. St Louis (MO): Mosby; 1998. p. 910–20.

20. Akoglu E, Karazincir S, Balci A, et al. Evaluation of the turbinate hypertrophy by computed tomography in patients with deviated nasal septum. Otolaryngol Head Neck Surg 2007;136:380–4.

21. Cook PR. Sinusitis and allergy. Curr Opin Otolaryngol 1997;5:35.

22. Baker DC. Treatment of obstructive inferior turbinates with intranasal corticosteroids. Ann Plast Surg 1979;3:253–9.

23. Mabry RL. Corticosteroids in otolaryngology: intraturbinal injection. Otolaryngol Head Neck Surg 1983;91:717–20.

24. Benninger M, Farrar JR, Blaiss M, et al. Evaluating approved medications to treat allergic rhinitis in the United States: an evidence-based review of efficacy for nasal symptoms by class. Ann Allergy Asthma Immunol 2010;104:13–29.

25. Carr WW, Ratner P, Munzel U, et al. Comparison of intranasal azelastine to intranasal fluticasone propionate for symptom control in moderate-to-severe seasonal allergic rhinitis. Allergy Asthma Proc 2012;33:450–8.

26. Poetker DM, Smith TL. Medicolegal implications of common rhinologic medications. Otolaryngol Clin North Am 2015;48:817–26.

27. Moss WJ, Lemieux AJ, Alexander TH. Is inferior turbinate lateralization effective? (letter). Plast Reconstr Surg 2015;136:710e–1e.

28. Jackson LE, Koch RJ. Controversies in the management of inferior turbinate hypertrophy: a comprehensive review. Plast Reconstr Surg 1999;103:300–12.

29. Aksoy F, Yildirim YS, Veyseller B, et al. Midterm outcomes of outfracture of the inferior turbinate. Otolaryngol Head Neck Surg 2010;143:579–84.

30. Passali D, Passali FM, Damiani V, et al. Treatment of inferior turbinate hypertrophy: a randomized clinical trial. Ann Otol Rhinol Laryngol 2003;112:683–8.

31. Assanasen P, Tantilipikorn P, Bunnag C. Combined microdebrider-assisted inferior turbinoplasty and lateral outfracture of hypertrophic inferior turbinate in the treatment of chronic rhinitis: short-term and long-term outcome. Asian Rhinol J 2015;2:63–5.

32. Rohrich RJ, Krueger JK, Adams WP, et al. Rationale for submucous resection of hypertrophied inferior turbinates in rhinoplasty: an evolution. Plast Reconstr Surg 2001;108:536–44.

33. Tsakiropoulou E, Vital V, Constantinidis J, et al. Nasal air-conditioning after partial turbinectomy: myths versus facts. Am J Rhinol Allergy 2015;29:e59–62.

34. Ishida H, Yoshida T, Hasegawa T, et al. Submucous electrocautery following submucous resection of turbinate bone—a rationale of surgical treatment for allergic rhinitis. Auris Nasus Larynx 2003;30:147–52.

35. Karlsson TR, Shakeel M, Supriya M, et al. Septoplasty with concomitant inferior turbinate reduction reduces the need for revision procedure. Rhinology 2015;53:59–65.

36. Becker SS, Dobratz EJ, Stowell N, et al. Revision septoplasty: review of sources of persistent nasal obstruction. Am J Rhinol 2008;22:440–4.

37. Han JK, Stringer SP, Rosenfeld RM, et al. Clinical consensus statement: septoplasty with or without inferior turbinate reduction. Otolaryngol Head Neck Surg 2015;153:708–20.

38. Moore GF, Freeman TJ, Ogren FP. Extended follow-up of total inferior turbinate resection for relief of chronic nasal obstruction. Laryngoscope 1985;95:1095–9.

39. Talmon Y, Samet A, Gilbey P. Total inferior turbinectomy: operative results and technique. Ann Otol Rhinol Laryngol 2000;109:1117–9.

40. Movahed R, Morales-Ryan C, Allen WR. Outcome assessment of 603 cases of concomitant inferior turbinectomy and Le Fort I osteotomy. Proc (Bayl Univ Med Cent) 2013;26:376–81.

41. Li KK, Powell NB, Riley RW. Radiofrequency volumetric tissue reduction for treatment of turbinate hypertrophy: a pilot study. Otolaryngol Head Neck Surg 1998;119:569–73.

42. Farmer SEJ, Eccles R. Understanding submucosal electrosurgery for the treatment of nasal turbinate enlargement. J Laryngol Otol 2007;121:615–21.

43. Gindros G, Kantas I, Balatsouras DG, et al. Comparison of ultrasound turbinate reduction, radiofrequency tissue ablation and submucosal cauterization in inferior turbinate hypertrophy. Eur Arch Otorhinolaryngol 2010;267:1727–33.

44. Mabry RL. Inferior turbinoplasty: patient selection, technique, and long-term consequences. Otolaryngol Head Neck Surg 1998;98:60.

45. Jose J, Coatesworth AP. Inferior turbinate surgery for nasal obstruction in allergic rhinitis after failed medical treatment. Cochrane Database Syst Rev 2010;(12):CD005235.

46. Stewart MG, Witsell DL, Smith TL, et al. Development and validation of the Nasal Obstruction Symptom Evaluation (NOSE) scale. Otolaryngol Head Neck Surg 2004;130:157–63.

47. Hwang SH, Kim SY, Park SH, et al. Human inferior turbinate: an alternative tissue source of multipotent mesenchymal stromal cells. Otolaryngol Head Neck Surg 2012;147:568–74.

48. Hwang SH, Park SH, Choi J, et al. Characteristics of mesenchymal stem cells originating from the bilateral inferior turbinate in humans with nasal septal deviation. PLoS One 2014;9:1–7.

The External Nasal Valve

Grant S. Hamilton III, MD

KEYWORDS

- External nasal valve • Nasal valve collapse • Batten graft • Nasal obstruction • Rhinoplasty
- Functional rhinoplasty • Nasal surgery • Septoplasty

KEY POINTS

- Nasal obstruction has a negative effect on quality of life. The external nasal valve plays an important role in nasal breathing and, consequently, nasal obstruction.
- Multiple anatomic structures make up the external nasal valve. Surgery to correct external nasal valve pathologic conditions must be tailored to the specific needs of the patient.
- A detailed understanding of the anatomy of the lower third of the nose is critical to proper treatment. Knowing how the anatomy contributes to pathologic conditions is as important as where it is.
- There are effective surgical and nonsurgical treatments for external nasal valve dysfunction.
- The muscles of the nose may play a bigger role in external nasal valve problems than is typically recognized.

Because the internal nasal valve has been identified as the narrowest segment in the nasal cavity, more has been written about the internal nasal valve than the external. A PubMed search at the time of this writing shows 202 articles when searching for "internal nasal valve" and 156 for "external nasal valve." However, the external nasal valve is the gateway to the nose. Pathologic conditions in the external valve are a complex interplay between the cartilage, skin, nasal muscles, vibrissae, and even the force of inspiration. This article aims to consolidate much of the current knowledge of external nasal valve problems and their treatment.

ANATOMY

Mink[1] was the first to identify the nasal valve as a single entity in 1903. To this day, in some articles, there is no differentiation between the internal nasal valve and the external nasal valve. Constantian and Martin[2] rightfully assert that this lack of consensus probably hinders rhinoplasty education. Distinguishing the internal from the external valve is important because they are distinct anatomic areas, though they do share a common border at the scroll. Many investigators describe the external nasal valve as the nostril opening; however, it is more clinically helpful to consider the nostril opening as a component of the external nasal valve.[3–5] In other words, the nostril opening is an area, whereas the external nasal valve is a volume. The borders of this space are the nostril opening caudally, the septum and medial crura medially, the alar cartilage and fibrofatty tissue anterolaterally, and the internal nasal valve opening posteriorly. With this many structures playing an important role in the integrity of the external nasal valve, it should be no surprise that there are multiple ways that external nasal valve insufficiency can manifest. Further complicating matters is that external nasal valve problems may be static, dynamic, or both.

The alar lobule is the convexity that abuts the cheek at the alar-facial junction, bordered superiorly by the alar groove. This curves medially, ending in a concavity posterior to the nasal tip lobule (**Fig. 1**). Ali-Salaam and colleagues[6] sectioned 15 cadavers and found that the alar lobule was devoid of cartilage in all specimens. The alar lobule is composed of skin, fibrofatty

Disclosure Statement: Spirox, Inc (consulting); no conflict of interest.
Department of Otorhinolaryngology, Mayo Clinic, 200 First Street SW, Rochester, MN 55905, USA
E-mail address: hamilton.grant@mayo.edu

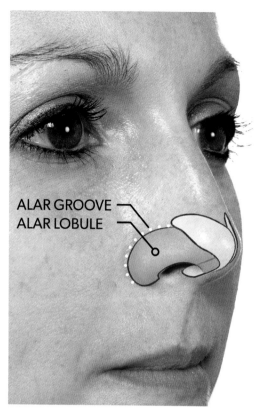

ALAR GROOVE
ALAR LOBULE

Fig. 1. The lower lateral cartilages are shown in white. The alar lobule is blue. The alar groove is the dotted line. Note that the lateral crura are not located in the alar lobule and that the point of maximal concavity of the alar groove is typically located at the lateral end of the lateral crus.

fascia, and muscle. The lateral crus travels superior to the alar groove and the investigators found that the lateral crura had 4 distinct anatomic variants. In some specimens, the lateral crus ended near the alar groove. In others, it continued along the alar groove and was either smooth or corrugated. Several had smaller, discontiguous sesamoid cartilages laterally.

The paired lower lateral cartilages are the primary structural component of the external nasal valve. Despite this, the alar cartilages are not usually as stiff as the septum. They begin medially at the feet of the medial crura. These are typically splayed somewhat from the midline. The medial crura sweep anterocephalically to the intermediate crura, where they twist laterally, creating a divergence in the area of the infratip lobule. The intermediate crura transition to the domes, a tighter bend that creates the definition of the tip. The domes should have an angle between them that is very obtuse. When the interdomal angle is too acute, the caudal margins of the lateral crura lie

closer to the septum. This has important implications for both form and function.[7] When the caudal edge of the lateral crus is close to the septum, the volume of the nasal vestibule is decreased. Aesthetically, this results in an alar rim that is poorly supported and will have a characteristic parenthesis deformity on the frontal view.

When describing the position of the lateral crus, it is helpful to think of it as having both a long and a short axis.[8] The long axis is a line that bisects the dome and roughly bisects the lateral crus along its length. The long axis should be oriented toward the lateral canthus.[9] When the long axis is positioned closer to the medial canthus, the lateral crura are said to be cephalically malpositioned. Cephalically malpositioned lateral crura are a significant contributor to external nasal valve incompetence. In a study by Constantian,[9] all secondary rhinoplasty patients in the sample who had cephalically malpositioned lateral crura had external nasal valve incompetence.

The short axis is perpendicular to the long axis and extends from the cephalic border of the lateral crus to the caudal border. Ideally, the short axis makes nearly a 90° angle with the septum.[7] When the angle between the septum and the short axis becomes more acute, the lateral crura are sagittally malpositioned and the vestibular volume is decreased. **Fig. 2** shows the relationships between the septum, dome angles, and the short and long axes of the lateral crura. Sagittally malpositioned lateral crura are also prone to acting like a hinge, predisposing to collapse of the valve.

Ideally, the shape of the lateral crus should be gently convex or flat. Markedly convex lateral crura will create a bulbous tip and will often be internally recurvate. Internally recurvate lateral crura create a mass effect in the nasal vestibule because the tail of the lateral crus is positioned too far medially toward the septum (**Fig. 3**). Concave lateral crura also decrease the volume of the external nasal valve and can lead to nasal obstruction.

The caudal septum should lie in a midsagittal plane between the medial crura. Therefore, the medial crura typically affect the nostril opening more than the caudal septum. Short or flared medial crura will widen the columella and subsequently narrow the nostril (**Fig. 4**). However, in patients with a severe caudal septal deflection, it may lie laterally to the medial crura and become the medial border of the nostril (**Fig. 5**).

The circumference of the external nasal valve, with the exception of the thin skin under the lateral crus and the mucosa of the septum, is lined with hair-bearing skin. Though the vibrissae have

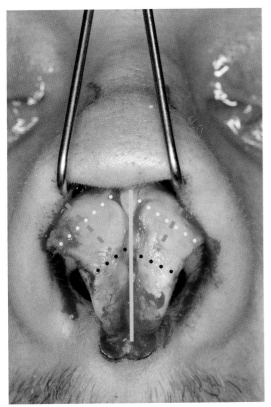

Fig. 2. The dome angles are represented by the black dotted lines. The short axes of the lateral crura are the yellow dotted lines. Note that they are parallel to the dome angles. Modifying the dome angles is an important component of repositioning the short axis of the lateral crus. The long axes of the lateral crura are represented by the green dashed lines.

an important job filtering out larger airborne particles, they have recently been shown to make a significant contribution to resistance in the external nasal valve.[10]

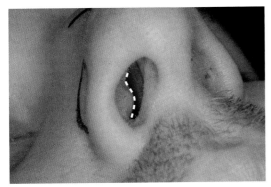

Fig. 3. When the lateral end of the lateral crus is internally recurvate, it obstructs the airway by impinging on the external nasal valve.

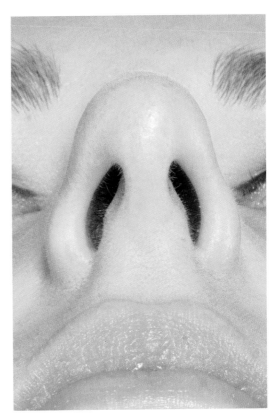

Fig. 4. Short medial crura create a widened columella, which narrows the nostrils and can lead to nasal obstruction.

Externally, the region of the external nasal valve is covered with skin. Under the skin are several important muscles of facial expression that affect the rigidity of the external nasal valve. Though Henry Gray[11] first described the nasal muscles in 1858, they are often overlooked in typical texts and lectures about rhinoplasty. One reason that these muscles may be less frequently discussed is that there is little agreement on concepts as basic as their names.[12–14] In an effort to clarify descriptions of the muscles in this article, alternate, typically older, names will be placed in parentheses.

The nasalis muscle (compressor nasi, musculus transversus) originates from the maxilla near the canine fossa and divides into a transverse and an alar part (dilator naris posterior, pars alaris). The transverse nasalis spans the dorsum and contracts the nostrils and compresses the nose. Its contraction narrows the external nasal valve. The alar part inserts onto the surface of the lateral crus and assists in dilating and stiffening the alar lobule.[12,15]

The musculus myrtiformis (musculus depressor septi nasi) also has 2 parts and originates near the

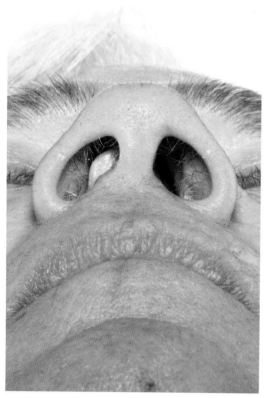

Fig. 5. A significant caudal septal deviation can also obstruct the external nasal valve.

nasalis on the maxilla near the canine fossa. The medial part inserts onto the caudal septum and medial crura. It is often referred to as the musculus depressor septi nasi and is responsible for depressing the nasal tip. The lateral part (depressor alae nasi) surrounds the nostril opening and opposes the lifting forces of the levator labii superioris alequae nasi and depresses and dilates the nostril.[12,15]

Similarly, the musculus procerus (musculus pyramidalis nasi) has 2 parts. It is located at the root of the nose between the eyebrows. The glabellar part joins with the transverse part of the nasalis and is primarily responsible for moving the medial eyebrow inferiorly. The alar part originates from the nasal bones and upper lateral cartilages, and inserts into the cephalic edge of the lateral crus and continues into the alar lobule. Its function is to elevate and dilate the alar rim.[12,15]

The levator labii superioris alequae nasi (caput angulare musculi quadrati labii superioris) inserts superiorly at the medial canthus, frontal process of the maxilla, and the nasal bones. It also divides into 2 parts. The alar part inserts on the cephalic border of the lateral crus and interdigitates with the alar part of the nasalis muscle. It elevates

and dilates the nostril. The labial fascicle joins the musculus myrtiformis and orbicularis oris, and contributes to the nasal tip depressors.[12]

Though originally described by Gray[11] in the first edition of his text, there has been disagreement from subsequent investigators about the exact location of the musculus anomalous nasi (musculus rhomboideus). Figallo and Acosta[12] describe it as a transverse muscle between the alar part of the procerus and the alar fascicle of the levator labii superioris alequae nasi. As it intermingles with the fibers of these muscles, it assists with elevation of the alar margin.[12,15]

The musculus dilator naris anterior (apices nasi) and the musculus compressor narium minor are in close apposition to the lower lateral cartilages, and play an important role in compressing the alae[12] **Table 1** summarizes the locations and functions of the previously described clinically relevant muscles.

Fig. 6 shows the effects of the muscles that insert into the external nasal valve. This patient had significant alar retraction and compression of the alar groove before surgery, in part due to excessive tone of his alar nasal musculature. **Fig. 6**A shows his nose before any intervention. Before his operation, he was treated with 10 units of onabotulinumtoxinA into each alar margin. His lateral nasal wall was reinforced with lateral crural strut grafts extending into the area of the alar groove during surgery. He declined any further chemodenervation treatment and is shown 2 weeks, 3 months, and 1 year after surgery. Despite the reinforcement of his lateral nasal wall with the lateral crural strut grafts, his alae returned to nearly their preoperative state.

Though some investigators have described the nasal muscles as rudimentary, as muscles of facial expression controlled by the facial nerve, the nasal musculature may be more voluntary and more integral to nasal breathing than typically thought. Vaiman and colleagues[16,17] performed several studies demonstrating the efficacy of treating nasal valve weakness with biofeedback via surface electromyography (EMG) with and without transcutaneous electrical stimulation of the nasal muscles. Aksoy and colleagues[18] specifically examined the role that the nasal muscles play in nasal valve dysfunction. When patients with dynamic nasal valve collapse were compared with healthy volunteers, those with collapse had statistically significant abnormalities in their use of musculus dilator naris anterior and the transverse part of the nasalis muscle during inspiration. Researchers at the Mayo Clinic measured both patency of the airway with rhinomanometry and alar stiffness in healthy volunteers. Measurements were taken before and after induced

Table 1
Nasal muscles

Muscle	Function
Musculus procerus (musculus pyramidalis nasi)	
Glabellar part	Moves the medial eyebrow inferiorly
Alar part	Elevates the alar rim and dilates the nostril
Levator labii superioris alequae nasi (caput angulare musculi quadrati labii superioris)	
Alar part	Elevates the alar rim and dilates the nostril
Labial part	With musculus myrtiformis depresses the nasal tip
Musculus anomalous nasi (musculus rhomboideus)	Elevates alar rim with levator labii superioris alequae nasi and procerus
Nasalis muscle (compressor nasi, musculus transversus)	
Transverse part	Narrows the external nasal valve
Alar part (dilator naris posterior, pars alaris)	Dilates and stiffens the alar lobule
Musculus myrtiformis	
Medial part (musculus depressor septi nasi)	Depresses the nasal tip
Lateral part (depressor alae nasi)	Depresses and dilates the nostril
Musculus dilator naris anterior (apices nasi)	Compresses the ala
Musculus compressor narium minor	Compresses the ala

muscular paresis with lidocaine. There was a statistically significant change after the injection, supporting their hypothesis that the nasal muscles make an important contribution to the patency of the airway.[19]

PHYSIOLOGY

The physiology of the external nose approximates that of a Starling resistor. Invented by Ernest Starling, a Starling resistor is a rigid tube with a collapsible segment controlled by changes in external pressure.[20] By changing the external pressure, Starling was able to simulate changes in peripheral vascular resistance. Similarly, during inspiration, a pressure gradient is created between the nasopharynx and the atmosphere. The deformable cartilaginous part of the external nose has a negative intraluminal pressure as a result of Bernoulli's principle: as the velocity of a fluid increases, its pressure decreases. Because the total flow of air must be equal at each end of a tube, its velocity must increase when passing through a narrowed segment, in this case, the internal and external nasal valves.[5] Poiseuille's Law is a tool that permits quantification of Bernoulli's principle. It states that the flow through a tube is proportional to the pressure differential multiplied by the radius of the tube raised to the fourth power. Consequently, small changes in the radius in either direction have a great impact on the flow.[5]

As the pressure differential between the inspired and extranasal air increases, the more flexible parts of the external nasal valve are prone to collapse; namely, the lateral wall. Rhee and Kimbell[21] summarize the problem of valve insufficiency as a problem of the opening being too narrow, the lateral wall being inadequately rigid, or both. Correction of nasal valve obstruction depends on accurate diagnosis of the underlying problem. Is it a static obstruction (septal deviation, internal recurvature of the lateral crus, widened columella, sagittally malpositioned lateral crura) or is it dynamic (cephalically malpositioned lateral crura, facial weakness)? Only by correctly identifying all the contributing factors can the surgeon adequately address the patient's concerns.

Airflow through the nose while breathing quietly is nearly laminar but becomes more turbulent as its velocity increases. Most inspired air travels through the middle meatus with smaller amounts above and below.[5] As people age, the nasal tip loses support and becomes ptotic. The counter-rotation of the tip alters the orientation of the nostril opening and directs the inspired air more cephalically, resulting in an increased work of breathing.[22] Slightly elevating the nasal tip during the examination can be a helpful diagnostic tool when identifying tip ptosis as the source of nasal obstruction in patients both young and old.

ANALYSIS

The history and physical examination are the foundation for identifying the source of external nasal

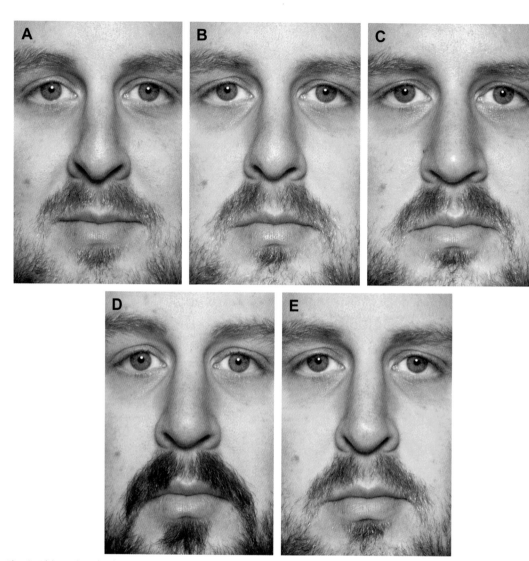

Fig. 6. This patient had nasal obstruction in part due to external nasal valve insufficiency. He had hypertonic nasal valve compressors before surgery. (*A*) Nose before any intervention. (*B*) Nose after treatment with 10 units of ona-botulinumtoxinA. Note that his alar retraction and nasal sidewall pinching is already improved. (*C*) The combined effects of onabotulinumtoxinA and lateral crural strut grafts 2 weeks after surgery. There is further improvement in the shape of his nasal alae and lateral nasal walls. (*D*) Three months after surgery. At this point, the effects of the onabotulinumtoxinA are gone. His alae are retracting and his sidewall becoming more pinched. (*E*) One year after surgery without any further onabotulinumtoxinA treatments. Though his breathing has improved, his nasal muscles have returned the shape of his nose to approximately its preoperative state.

valve dysfunction. While taking the history, watch how the patient breathes. Is there collapse during quiet respiration or does the patient need to demonstrate it with a vigorous breath in? Some patients occlude 1 nostril at a time to identify the side of obstruction. Many times when doing this they push hard enough that the caudal septum and columella shift onto the contralateral nostril, causing obstruction there too. This activity should be discouraged. If patients persist in using this

technique to assess their nasal breathing after surgery, it will be nearly impossible to satisfy them. Do they volunteer that a Cottle maneuver improves their symptoms? Patients who have discovered this will often sleep in such a way that their pillow will put traction on their cheek. Ask if they have tried external or internal splinting devices. This is a good indicator that the problem is due, at least in part, to the external nasal valve. If the patient has glasses, ask them to try them on. Heavy eyeglasses may slide down the nose and pinch the lateral nasal wall.

During the physical examination, first inspect the nose. Patients with external nasal valve dysfunction will often have 1 or more characteristic findings on examination. Thick, sebaceous skin may be harder to support laterally. A deep alar groove may signify internal recurvature of the lateral crus. A parenthesis deformity of the tip typically represents an underlying sagittal malposition of the lateral crus. These patients will often have slit-like nostrils but this is not pathognomonic. Narrow nostrils are also often present in patients who are overprojected. A bulbous tip and alar retraction are often found when the lateral crura are cephalically malpositioned. A widened columella from short medial crura will narrow the nostril openings causing both a static and dynamic obstruction. If the patient is ultimately a candidate for surgery, short medial crura should prompt some measure to support the base of the nose. Thick vibrissae can cause a significant increase in the work of breathing.[10] Look for asymmetry of the medial crura. This almost always indicates a deviation of the caudal septum. Does the patient seem to be inadvertently pinching the valve in the alar groove due to hypertonicity of the nasal muscles? Blanching of the alar rim may be a clue that the alar compressors are overactive. Conversely, examine the patient's facial nerve function. Facial weakness affecting the nasal musculature often results in nasal obstruction from an inability to tense and dilate the lateral nasal wall.[23,24]

Next, have the patient look at the ceiling. First ask them to take a typical breath in and look for collapse. Repeat this with a more forceful inspiration. When doing this, be aware that in patients who have an anterior septal deviation impinging on the nasal vestibule, the contralateral external valve may collapse with deep inspiration. If this happens, look critically for other causes of external valve insufficiency. It may be that the lateral wall is moving inward only because that nostril is doing the work of 2, with a concomitant increase in airflow and decrease in intraluminal pressure. If no other cause of lateral wall weakness can be identified, a septoplasty may be the only surgery needed.[25]

Less commonly, scarring can cause a circumferential contracture of the external nasal valve. This is a challenging problem beyond the scope of this article. Successful treatment of the stenotic nasal vestibule usually mandates cicatricial excision, dilation, and grafting.[26]

Next palpate the nose. Is the tip easily compressible? A missed diagnosis of a poorly supported nasal base will predispose the patient to postoperative tip ptosis and nasal obstruction. In a patient with ptosis, lift the tip to approximate a realistic surgical outcome and ask the patient if this improves their symptoms. Next, gently palpate the lateral nasal walls and the lateral crura to feel how rigid they are. In my experience, a standard Cottle maneuver (lateral traction on the cheek, near the alar groove) is of little diagnostic value because patients without nasal obstruction feel that it improves their nasal breathing. Also, unless one is planning to place a lateral traction suture in the cheek, the Cottle maneuver does not approximate anything offered by standard rhinoplasty techniques. However, a modified Cottle maneuver can be a very valuable diagnostic technique.[27] Some investigators advocate using a cotton-tipped swab to support the external nasal valve. This has the disadvantage that the swab itself occupies a significant amount of space in the nasal vestibule. Alternately, a small ear curette takes up almost no space in the nose and can precisely target the area to be affected most by surgery, giving a reasonable approximation of the outcome. This is helpful information when deciding whether or not the patient will perceive a benefit from surgery. Keep in mind that this simulation cannot account for other causes of obstruction, such as a deformed septum, and may limit the patient's ability to appreciate the improvement from the modified Cottle maneuver alone. Poirrier and colleagues[28] have developed a validated grading scale for assessing the severity of external nasal valve collapse that may be useful for surgical planning and evaluation of surgical outcomes. Each nostril is evaluated independently and scored from 0 to 2 (0 = no movement, 2 = complete collapse) during gentle and deep inspiration. This gives a total possible score between 0 and 4 for each side. Bohluli and colleagues[29] propose a similar solution using software to compare the area on standardized photographs of the base of the nose. Tools like these are important for outcomes research in the context of evidence-based medicine.

Use a speculum and a bright light to examine the anterior nasal passages. Look for septal deviations that impinge on the external nasal valve. On the lateral wall, internally recurvate lateral crura will be evident as a bump at the tail of the lateral crus (see **Fig. 3**). Follow this with a flexible or rigid endoscopic examination of the remainder of the nasal cavity. Note that the evaluation previously described only applies to the external nasal valve and is only a portion of a thorough nasal examination.

MEASUREMENT

Objective measurement of external nasal valve patency is a challenging endeavor due to the limitations of the tests and the problem of the test interfering with the results. Acoustic rhinometry can measure the volume of the nasal passage but will not account for the dynamic nature of valve collapse. Placement of masks for rhinomanometry may stent the valve similar to a Cottle maneuver, thereby creating an artificially improved airway. Similarly, any probes placed in the nose may act as stents themselves.[30] Validated scales (previously detailed), standardized photographs, and patient-reported outcome measurements are the most clinically useful measures of external nasal valve insufficiency.

NONSURGICAL TREATMENT

There are several inexpensive commercial devices that will stent the external nasal valve in patients who are poor candidates for surgery (**Fig. 7**). External nasal dilators such as Breathe Right nasal strips (GlaxoSmithKline, 980 Great West Road, Brentford, Middlesex, TW8 9GS, UK) work by stiffening and expanding the lateral nasal wall. In a thorough review from 2014, Reis Dinardi and colleagues[31] concluded that external nasal dilators are well tolerated and favorably affect the area of the nasal valve, nasal resistance, and lateral wall stability. However, they did state that more studies are needed, especially in children.

Internal nasal dilators are also effective nonsurgical alternatives. Hellings and Nolst Trenité[32] tested the Airmax (Airmax BV, Rhijngeesterstraatweg 58A, 2341 BV Oegstgeest, The Netherlands) nasal dilator in 30 subjects with bilateral external nasal valve dysfunction. They found that the

mean peak nasal inspiratory flow in their subjects increased by 176.1% plus or minus 59.6%. Although 11 out of 30 subjects discontinued use of the Airmax after the conclusion of the study, they did so for reasons unrelated to the effectiveness of the device. Multiple studies have demonstrated that internal and external nasal dilators are a safe, inexpensive, and effective way to treat external nasal valve dysfunction without surgery.

Stoddard and colleagues[10] studied, for the first time, the effect of the vibrissae on both subjective and objective measurements of nasal obstruction. Thirty subjects without symptoms of nasal obstruction were stratified into 3 groups based on the density of their vibrissae. Before rhinomanometric measurement, the subjects were decongested to minimize the contribution of the mucosa to their nasal resistance. Subjective measurements were then taken using a modified Nasal Obstruction Symptom Evaluation (NOSE) scale and objective measurements using a full-face mask rhinomanometer to prevent an unwanted Cottle maneuver from the mask. The vibrissae were trimmed and both measurements were repeated. The participants with denser vibrissae noted a statistically significant improvement in both NOSE scores and rhinomanometric measurements. Based on these data, the vibrissae are a previously unstudied resistor in the external nasal valve. Trimming the vibrissae in patients with moderate or many nasal hairs is a low-risk, inexpensive way to improve nasal breathing.

Vaiman and colleagues[16,17] performed 2 studies investigating the effectiveness of biofeedback combined with a home exercise program to train patients to better support the lateral nasal wall musculature. In 2005, they studied 15 people with symptomatic nasal obstruction due to nasal valve collapse. They were treated with a specific course of exercises combined with intranasal and surface EMG to provide biofeedback. They found that 86% of the patients had a significant enough subjective and objective improvement that they no longer needed surgery. Similar results were found in the study from 2004. This type of physical therapy may benefit patients who are unable or unwilling to have surgery but it is unclear if exercises alone are of benefit. However, if EMG biofeedback is required for successful treatment, widespread adoption of these techniques may be limited.

Nonsurgical treatments for external nasal valve insufficiency include

- Internal or external vestibular splints
- Trim the vibrissae
- Physical therapy to improve muscular stenting of the valve.

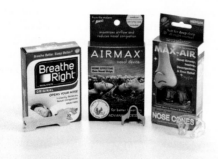

Fig. 7. A selection of commercially available internal and external nasal dilators. Breathe Right (Philadelphia Navy Yard, Philadelphia, PA, USA); Air Max (McKeon Products, Inc, Warren, MI, USA); Max Air (Sanostec Corp, Beverly Farms, MA, USA).

SURGICAL TECHNIQUES
Caudal Septal Deformities

The caudal septum is easily displaced from the anterior nasal spine and, because of its position, is particularly vulnerable to trauma. Because it cannot simply be removed, straightening the caudal septum is the most challenging part of a septoplasty. Straightening the caudal septum with any method can be accomplished through either an endonasal or external approach. When the caudal septum is flat but displaced from the maxillary crest, a swinging door technique can be used to reposition the caudal septum on the anterior nasal spine, typically held in place with a suture.[5] If the spine is not in the midline, the septum can be placed in a groove on the contralateral side of the spine and sutured to it. Sometimes, a gentle caudal septal deflection can be corrected by elevating the mucoperichondrium completely and skeletonizing the caudal septum. It is important to understand why the caudal septum is bent. It may be inherently curved but, not infrequently, the septum is too tall and curves to fit in the nose. Resecting a small amount of cartilage from the inferior part of the caudal septum may permit the cartilage to stand straighter.[33]

Some surgeons advocate scoring the cartilage on the concave side to relax intrinsic stresses in the septum. Though this can be effective, I find this unreliable when used alone. Splinting the septum with cartilage or thin bone on the scored side makes for a more reliable repair (**Fig. 8**). Wee and colleagues[33] studied 30 subjects who received septal batten grafts of cartilage or bone. In their series, 90% of the subjects had a straight septum postoperatively but all of them had improvements in their NOSE scores. There was also a statistically significant difference in the mean minimal cross-sectional area and the nasal volume when measured with acoustic rhinometry.

When the caudal septum is too weak or deformed to be repositioned or reinforced, it should be resected and replaced. In a primary septoplasty patient there is usually adequate tissue in the central part of the quadrangular cartilage to make a caudal septal replacement graft. Make certain to leave a strong attachment to the ethmoid bone at the keystone area by redirecting the chondrotomy to a more posterior direction[34] (**Fig. 9**). After the cartilage is removed, measure the distance from the anterior nasal spine to the anterior septal angle. Use this as the critical dimension when designing a caudal septal replacement graft. The graft should be at least 1 cm in depth, 1 to 2 mm wide and is typically 2.5 cm tall. Use a 4-0 polydioxanone suture to affix the graft to the anterior nasal spine and rotate it into position at the anterior end of the dorsal strut. Attach the graft to the dorsal strut with at least 3 5-0 polydioxanone sutures arranged in a triangle. This will prevent the graft from hinging or pivoting.[35]

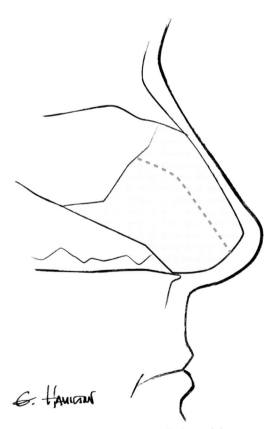

Fig. 9. When replacing a crooked caudal septum, leave a significant attachment at the ethmoid bone by curving the chondrotomy posteriorly as it approaches the keystone area.

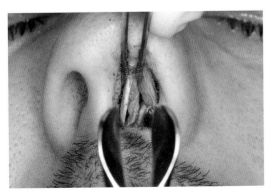

Fig. 8. A septal batten graft being placed endonasally to straighten the caudal septum.

Options for correcting caudal septal deflections include

- Reposition in the midline
- Reinforce with a septal batten graft
- Replace the crooked caudal septum with straight cartilage.

Tip Ptosis

When the nasal tip is ptotic, it is may be necessary to support the nasal base to increase rotation. Techniques for strengthening the nasal base include the columellar strut, caudal septal extension graft, caudal septal replacement graft, and suturing the medial crura to the caudal septum.[7] Though the columellar strut is commonly used to support the nasal base, it is more predictably used for increasing projection, not rotation. To rotate the nose with more precision, consider another method in which the medial crura are sutured to the septum. If using a caudal extension or caudal replacement graft, it should be somewhat wider at the base than at the tip to allow the lower lateral cartilages to rotate cephalically.

If the tip needs to be rotated and deprojected at the same time, dividing and overlapping the lateral crura will accomplish both goals. This can be done endonasally or through an external approach. If using an endonasal approach, make a marginal incision. Next, hydrodissect the vestibular skin from the undersurface of the lateral crus with local anesthesia. Mark a spot several millimeters lateral to the dome. Then, estimate the amount of overlap needed and make a second mark. Elevate the vestibular skin from the lateral crus, being careful not to tear the skin. Divide the lateral crura

transversely at the first mark and overlap the medial part over the lateral segment. Affix it with a 5-0 polydioxanone suture.[36] The amount of overlap can be adjusted to account for asymmetries in the lateral crura.

Sinno and colleagues[37] recently performed a review of the literature regarding the effectiveness of disrupting the depressor septi nasi muscle. They reviewed 19 studies and found that, although there was some variation in the anatomic description of the muscle, the consensus in the literature is that disrupting the depressor septi nasi muscle has a beneficial effect on tip ptosis.

Deprojection

When patients are overprojected and have narrow nostrils, deprojecting the nose will cause the nostrils to flare, increasing the area of the nostril opening. Because of the shape of the caudal septum, deprojecting the nose is especially suited to affixing the medial crura to the septum in a tongue-in-groove manner. Doing so will help prevent unintended counter-rotation. Whether using an endonasal or external approach, it is necessary to free all the attachments to the caudal septum to permit a complete release of the tip. Patients with a tension nose deformity will often have narrow nostrils and short medial crura. After deprojection, the feet of the medial crura will be closer to the lip, narrowing the columella and further opening the nostril (**Fig. 10**).

Batten Grafts

Free-floating batten grafts are an easy way to reinforce a weak lateral nasal wall. However, because

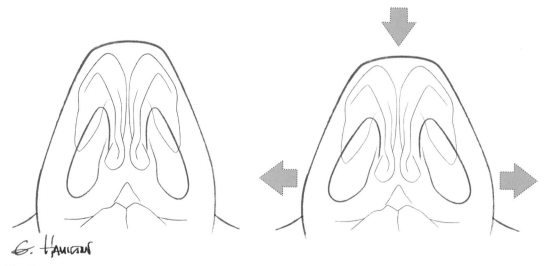

Fig. 10. Deprojecting the nose has the effect of flaring the nostrils and bringing the wide medial crural feet closer to the lip. These will both open the external nasal valve.

they add bulk, there is a risk of making the patient's obstruction worse if placed in the wrong candidate. A good candidate will have a reasonably open nasal vestibule that collapses with inspiration. Patients who have very narrow vestibules are at risk for worsening symptoms after batten graft placement (**Fig. 11**). When placing batten grafts for internal nasal valve collapse, they should be placed over the scroll.[38] For external valve collapse, they should be placed in line with or caudal to the lateral crus.[39] There is a lack of consensus about the importance of extending the graft to the piriform aperture.[39–41] I prefer not to extend them all the way to the bone, finding that doing so can create an unsightly fullness in the alar groove. A batten graft can be made of septal, conchal, or costal cartilage. Ideally, the cartilage should have a gentle curvature to it. Place the concavity of the cartilage toward the airway. When using costal cartilage, the fibrous, outer layer of the rib can be shaved to create an excellent batten graft. This type of graft is thin, elastic, and durable. In general, a batten graft should be 8 to 10 mm wide, 1.5 to 2.0 cm long, and 1 mm thick. It is helpful to taper it somewhat to facilitate insertion into a tight pocket in the lateral nasal wall.

Bevel the edges of the graft to decrease the probability of the graft being palpated by the patient. I mark the point of maximal concavity of the alar groove and use that as the target for graft placement. If the patient has internally recurvate lateral crura, the graft can be placed under the tail of the lateral crus to keep it out of the airway. It is important to make the pocket for the graft just deep to the vestibular skin. Making the pocket too close to the external skin may displace soft tissue into the airway and increase the likelihood of graft visibility. The external approach provides excellent access for placing an alar batten graft. Endonasal placement can also be accomplished through a marginal incision. I make a small backcut at the lateral end of the marginal incision to facilitate creation of the pocket and insertion of the graft (**Fig. 12**).

Lateral Crus Modification

There are many published techniques for modification of the lateral crura. Space does not permit an exhaustive review here. This discussion is limited to commonly used techniques that solve most problems of the lateral crus that relate to external

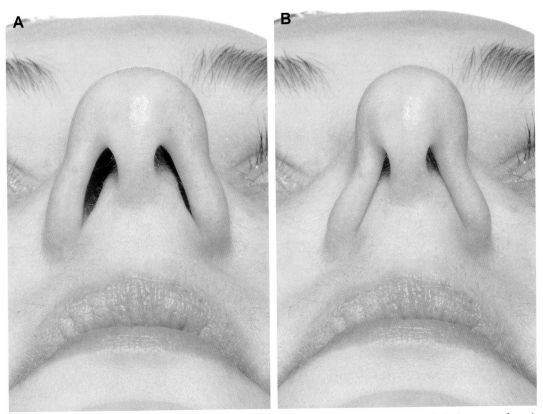

Fig. 11. This patient has very narrow nostrils and would likely be made worse by placement of alar batten grafts only. She needs columellar narrowing and reinforcement and repositioning of her lateral crura. (*A*) At rest. (*B*) Inspiration.

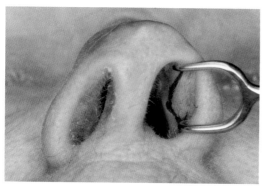

Fig. 12. When placing alar batten grafts endonasally, it is helpful to make a small back-cut to facilitate pocket development and graft insertion.

valve dysfunction. When evaluating the lateral crus, I find it helpful to identify whether there are problems of lateral crural position, lateral crural shape, or both. When the lateral crura are cephalically or sagittally malpositioned, the solution is to reorient them into a more anatomically appropriate position. Cephalic malposition is a problem of the long axis of the lateral crus, whereas sagittal malposition is a problem of the short axis **(Fig. 13)**. The most common way to address cephalically malpositioned lateral crura is to dissect them free from the vestibular skin, reinforce

them with lateral crural strut grafts, and reposition them into more caudally oriented pockets.[7,8,39,42] Unlike correction of cephalic malposition, correction of sagittally malpositioned lateral crura often requires more than 1 technique in the same patient. The goal of sagittal malposition correction is to elevate the caudal border of the lateral crus to approximately the same height as the cephalic border, making the short axis nearly perpendicular to the septum. To facilitate this rotation around the length of the lateral crus, it is helpful to perform a conservative cephalic trim. By releasing the lateral crus from the compound curve of the scroll, it is more easily reshaped and repositioned. Placing a dome suture to create a more favorable dome angle can elevate the caudal margin of the lateral crus.[8] In recalcitrant cases, a small wedge of cartilage can be removed from the cephalic edge of the dome to encourage a more horizontal orientation of the dome.[8] Note that an improperly placed single or double-dome suture can create or exacerbate the problem of the caudal edge of the lateral crus moving too close to the septum. Lee and Guyuron[43] have reported using subdomal grafts to successfully reorient the lateral crus to a more horizontal position. Lateral crural strut grafts and spanning sutures can also be used to reorient the lateral crura to be more perpendicular to the septum.[8]

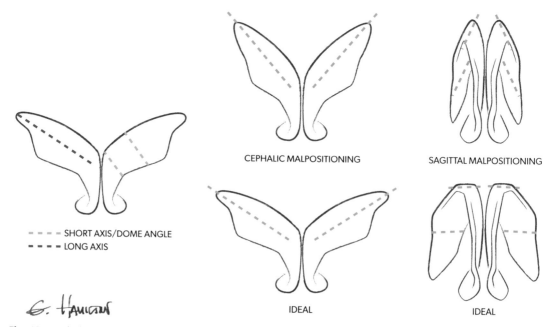

CEPHALIC MALPOSITIONING

SAGITTAL MALPOSITIONING

- - - - SHORT AXIS/DOME ANGLE
▬ ▬ ▬ LONG AXIS

IDEAL

IDEAL

Fig. 13. Cephalic malposition is a problem of the long axis of the lateral crus, whereas sagittal malposition is a problem of the short axis. The goal of sagittal malposition correction is to elevate the caudal border of the lateral crus to approximately the same height as the cephalic border, making the short axis nearly perpendicular to the septum. Note that the dome angle should be nearly perpendicular to the plane of the septum.

Deformities of the lateral crura are also a common problem. Lateral crural turn-in flaps are a straightforward way to flatten and strengthen the lateral crus.[39,44] These flaps are created by scoring the lateral crus along its length and folding the cephalic segment caudally into a pocket between the lateral crus and the vestibular skin. Sutures fix the 2 layers of cartilage together, creating a laminated structure. It is important to leave enough of a lateral crus to prevent postoperative alar retraction. Typically, 8 mm is a safe minimum.

Lateral crural strut grafts placed in pockets between the cartilage and vestibular skin are also a reliable way to flatten and reinforce the lateral crura.[7,8,39,44] When the lateral crura are concave, they can be excised lateral to the dome and swapped, flipping them over as they are transposed.[39,40] This expands the vestibular volume by turning the concavity into a convexity. A simultaneous turn-in flap can help to flatten the lateral crura if they are too convex. If the lateral crura are inadequate due to trauma or previous surgery, they may need to be excised lateral to the dome and replaced.

Alar Rim Grafts

Alar rim grafts are a good adjunctive technique for supporting the alar margin. It would be unlikely that a rim graft would be the entire solution to a patient's alar collapse but, in conjunction with other techniques described here, they can impart added strength to the alar rim.[39,45,46] Guyuron and colleagues[47] recently completed a study of 665 subjects who received alar rim grafts. They found that rim grafts were an effective way to reinforce the nostril margin, resulting in a smoother contour, increased cross-sectional area, and a caudal translocation of the alar rim.

Columellar Modification

When a wide columella is partially obstructing the nostrils, there are several options for narrowing it. One was discussed previously in the context of deprojecting the tip. If that is not indicated, the columellar base can be narrowed. Lawson and Reino[48] recommend excising a diamond of skin and soft tissue from between the medial crura and suturing the medial crural feet together. I use a similar technique. First mark a transverse line over each medial crural foot at the point of maximal flare. Next, mark a 2 mm midline incision on the columella at the level of the lateral markings. After infiltrating a small amount of local anesthetic, make a stab incision at the point marked on the columella. Using a fine forceps and scissors,

remove some soft tissue from between the medial crura through this small opening. With a 15 blade, incise the skin over the medial crural feet making sure not to cut the cartilage. Use a small scissor to elevate the skin for a couple of millimeters above and below these incisions. Pass a 4-0 clear nylon suture from the midline incision to the right medial crural incision at its anterior edge. Return the suture through the posterior part of the incision and pass it through to the posterior part of the left medial crural incision. Finally, pass the suture from the anterior part of the left medial crural incision back to the midline columellar incision. Pull the suture tight to see the effect of narrowing the columella. When the tension is right, place several knots and close the incisions with a 7-0 nylon suture.

Suspension Sutures

Suspension sutures are a minimally invasive way to support the lateral nasal wall. Several techniques have been described. Menger[49] developed a method of using a permanent suture to affix the tail of the lateral crus to the piriform aperture in a more cephalad position. Paniello[50] developed the technique of using a permanent suture to suspend the nasal valve from the inferior orbital rim, with good results. White and Hamilton[51] (latter is the current author) have recently described a technique using a bone-anchored, permanent suture from the malar eminence to the external nasal valve to pull in a more lateral direction, simulating a Cottle maneuver. Suture suspension of the lateral nasal wall has been shown to be a safe technique. I have found this especially useful in patients with facial paralysis due to their lack of dilatory muscle tone in the nostril.[24]

OUTCOMES

In 2003, Rhee and colleagues[52] performed a cross-sectional study to determine the preoperative quality of life (QOL) in patients with nasal obstruction and to identify the variables most predictive of their QOL and to correlate QOL measures with patient's self-assessments of their nasal obstruction. Forty patients with surgically correctable nasal obstruction were included. The Rhinoconjunctivitis Quality of Life Questionnaire and the Rhinosinusitis Disability Index were used as measurement tools. They found that patients who had nasal valve dysfunction felt more obstructed than those with septal deformities. In general, QOL was not correlated with physical examination findings but patients with both septal deviation and nasal valve dysfunction reported worse nasal obstruction than those with either septal or valve pathologic conditions alone.

Two years later, Rhee and colleagues[53] studied QOL improvements after nasal valve surgery in 26 subjects. In their multicenter study, they did not differentiate between internal and external nasal valve problems. They also included subjects with septal deviations and turbinate hypertrophy. Treatment was functional septorhinoplasty, which encompassed multiple modalities intended to correct deformities associated with nasal obstruction. The primary outcome measure was the NOSE scale. They also used a visual analog scale (VAS) that was completed by the surgeon grading the severity of nasal obstruction. They concluded that surgery of the nasal valve improved disease-specific QOL. In contrast to the study in 2003, the surgeon-rated VAS correlated with the patients' QOL, indicating that an experienced surgeon may be able to predict QOL improvements in patients.

Similarly, Chambers and colleagues[54] assessed improvement in 40 subjects with internal and/or external nasal valve obstruction after failed septoplasties. Outcomes were evaluated using the NOSE survey. In their sample, 18 out of 40 subjects had external nasal valve narrowing, whereas 16 out of 40 had external valve collapse. Additionally, 10 out of 40 subjects had flared medial crura, 5 out of 40 had internally recurvate lateral crura, and 7 out of 40 had cephalically malpositioned lateral crura. Subjects had surgery targeted to their specific valve problems using a variety of techniques. Spreader grafts and lateral crural strut grafts were the most common valve-specific interventions. Because the subjects in this study may have had multiple simultaneous valve problems, there is no way to quantify the success of the interventions targeted at only the external valve. Nevertheless, of the 33 out of 40 people who completed postoperative NOSE surveys, there was a statistically significant improvement.

Chung, Lee, and Scott[55] retrospectively investigated the effects of nasal valve surgery in 15 children under the age of 16 without cleft-related nasal deformities. Their series also included internal nasal valve repair with spreader grafts. Alar batten grafts were placed in 4 subjects and 1 received alar rim grafts. The outcome measure was documentation in the chart of subjects' satisfaction and a lack of complications. Though this was a short-term, retrospective study, all subjects studied were satisfied at 90 days and the only complication was a bout of self-limiting epistaxis.

In addition to Wee and colleagues[33] 2012 study on the success of septal batten grafting, Chung and colleagues[56] performed a study in 2014 investigating the utility of bony septal batten grafts to correct caudal septal deviations. Subjects used a VAS to assess 10 symptoms related to nasal obstruction. Acoustic rhinometry and evaluation of the minimum cross-sectional area of the convex side was also performed. Like Wee and colleagues,[33] they found an improvement using septal batten grafts to straighten the caudal septum.

Palesy and colleagues[57] recently compared subjective and objective measures of the outcome from surgery to correct the external nasal valve. They studied 19 subjects who had costal cartilage lateral crural strut grafts or cephalic turn-in flaps. Despite an insignificant change in the minimum cross-sectional area, they found an increase in peak nasal inspiratory flow and improvement in both the Sinonasal Outcome Test and the NOSE scale. They conclude that stiffening the lateral nasal wall improves external valve performance.

Silva Filho Rde and Pochat[58] performed a cadaver study in 2016 measuring the effects of lateral crural strut grafts on the shape of the external nasal valve. They performed lateral crural strut grafts in 16 cadavers and found statistically significant differences in basilar-nasal width, nostril cross-sectional area, and the height of the columella from the nasolabial angle to the tip. They conclude that the changes to the nostril cross-sectional area improve the patency of the external nasal valve.

Constantian and Clardy[59] completed a rigorous study of both the internal and external nasal valves. They prospectively evaluated 160 consecutive subjects without turbinate hypertrophy or septal perforation. Their airways were assessed by rhinomanometry before and after surgery, decongesting them beforehand to minimize any confounding mucosal effects. Surgically, subjects were treated with septoplasty, spreader, or dorsal grafts in the internal valve, and bone or cartilage grafts in the external valve. Subjects in this cohort who only had septal surgery had a statistically insignificant improvement in mean nasal airflow. In contrast, when subjects had surgery only on the external nasal valve, their airflow was 2.6 times greater. When subjects had both a septoplasty and external nasal valve reconstruction, their airflow was increased 4.9 times compared with their preoperative measurements. They also noted that 110 of the 160 subjects had unilateral obstructing symptoms. Somewhat surprisingly, only 46% of these subjects had a septal deviation toward the side of their symptoms. They concluded that, not only does the nasal valve play an important role in nasal breathing, its effects may be more clinically significant than that of a deviated septum.

SUMMARY

The external nasal valve is an entity that is still not well understood. No doubt this is because there still seems to be no consensus about what, exactly, it is. Also, there are relatively few studies that have investigated its contribution to nasal breathing independent from other important structures in the nose. Nevertheless, the data we do have are in agreement that the external nasal valve makes significant contributions to the nasal airway. In the future, I suspect that a better appreciation of the importance of the orientation of the lateral crus as opposed to only its location will be gained. Certainly there is fertile ground for further research.

REFERENCES

1. Mink PJ. Le nez comme voie respiratoire. Presse Otolaryngol 1903;481–96.
2. Constantian MB, Martin JP. Why can't more good surgeons learn rhinoplasty? Aesthet Surg J 2015; 35:486–9.
3. Lam SM, Williams EF. Anatomic considerations in aesthetic rhinoplasty. Facial Plast Surg 2002;18(4): 209–14.
4. Wulkan M, Julio de Andrade Sá A, Alonso N. Modified technique to increase nostril cross-sectional area after using rib and septal cartilage graft over alar nasal cartilages. Acta Cir Bras 2012;27:713–9.
5. Howard BK, Rohrich RJ. Understanding the nasal airway: principles and practice. Plast Reconstr Surg 2002;109:1128–46 [quiz: 1145–6].
6. Ali-Salaam P, Kashgarian M, Davila J, et al. Anatomy of the Caucasian alar groove. Plast Reconstr Surg 2002;110(1):261–6 [discussion: 267–71].
7. Toriumi DM. New concepts in nasal tip contouring. Arch Facial Plast Surg 2006;8(3):156–85.
8. Hamilton GS. Form and function of the nasal tip: reorienting and reshaping the lateral crus. Facial Plast Surg 2016;32(1):49–58.
9. Constantian MB. The boxy nasal tip, the ball tip, and alar cartilage malposition: variations on a theme—a study in 200 consecutive primary and secondary rhinoplasty patients. Plast Reconstr Surg 2005;116(1): 268–81.
10. Stoddard DG, Pallanch JF, Hamilton GS. The effect of vibrissae on subjective and objective measures of nasal obstruction. Am J Rhinol Allergy 2015;29: 373–7.
11. Gray H. Anatomy descriptive and surgical, vol. 1. England (United Kingdom): John William Parker and Son; 1858.
12. Figallo EE, Acosta JA. Nose muscular dynamics: the tip trigonum. Plast Reconstr Surg 2001;108(5): 1118–26.
13. Hoeyberghs JL, Desta K, Matthews RN. The lost muscles of the nose. Aesthet Plast Surg 1996; 20(2):165–9.
14. Zide BM. Nasal anatomy: the muscles and tip sensation. Aesthet Plast Surg 1985;9(3):193–6.
15. Guyuron B. Soft tissue functional anatomy of the nose. Aesthet Surg J 2006;26(6):733–5.
16. Vaiman M, Eviatar E, Segal S. Muscle-building therapy in treatment of nasal valve collapse. Rhinology 2004;42(3):145–52.
17. Vaiman M, Shlamkovich N, Kessler A, et al. Biofeedback training of nasal muscles using internal and external surface electromyography of the nose. Am J Otolaryngol 2005;26(5):302–7.
18. Aksoy F, Veyseller B, Yıldırım YS, et al. Role of nasal muscles in nasal valve collapse. Otolaryngol Head Neck Surg 2010;142(3):365–9.
19. Kienstra MA, Gassner HG, Sherris DA, et al. Effects of the nasal muscles on the nasal airway. Am J Rhinol 2005;19(4):375–81.
20. Knowlton FP, Starling EH. The influence of variations in temperature and blood-pressure on the performance of the isolated mammalian heart. J Physiol 1912;44:206–19.
21. Rhee JS, Kimbell JS. The nasal valve dilemma: the narrow straw vs the weak wall. Arch Facial Plast Surg 2012;14(1):9–10.
22. Rohrich RJ, Hollier LH, Janis JE, et al. Rhinoplasty with advancing age. Plast Reconstr Surg 2004;114: 1936–44.
23. Shindo M. Management of facial nerve paralysis. Otolaryngol Clin North Am 1999;32(5):945–64.
24. Kayabasoglu G, Nacar A. Secondary Improvement in static facial reanimation surgeries: increase of nasal function. J Craniofac Surg 2015;26(4): e335–337.
25. Schalek P, Hahn A. Anterior septal deviation and contralateral alar collapse. B-ENT 2011;7(3):185–8.
26. Daines SM, Hamilton GS, Mobley SR. A graded approach to repairing the stenotic nasal vestibule. Arch Facial Plast Surg 2010;12:332–8.
27. Fung E, Hong P, Moore C, et al. The effectiveness of modified cottle maneuver in predicting outcomes in functional rhinoplasty. Plast Surg Int 2014;2014(2): 1–6.
28. Poirrier AL, Ahluwalia S, Kwame I, et al. External nasal valve collapse: validation of novel outcome measurement tool. Rhinology 2014;52:127–32.
29. Bohluli B, Varedi P, Kahali R, et al. External nasal valve efficacy index: a simple test to evaluate the external nasal valve. Int J Oral Maxillofac Surg 2015;44(10):1240–5.
30. Kenyon GS. Objective measurement of the external nasal valve. Clin Otolaryngol 2015;40(1):67.
31. Reis Dinardi R, Ribeiro de Andrade C, da Cunha Ibiapina C. External nasal dilators: definition, background, and current uses. Int J Gen Med 2014;7:491.

32. Hellings PW, Nolst Trenité G. Improvement of nasal breathing and patient satisfaction by the endonasal dilator Airmax®. Rhinology 2014;52(1):31–4.

33. Wee JH, Lee J-E, Cho S-W, et al. Septal batten graft to correct cartilaginous deformities in endonasal septoplasty. Arch Otolaryngol Head Neck Surg 2012;138(5):457–61.

34. Mau T, Mau S-t, Kim DW. Cadaveric and engineering analysis of the septal L-strut. Laryngoscope 2007; 117(11):1902–6.

35. Wu PS, Hamilton GS. Extracorporeal septoplasty: external and endonasal techniques. Facial Plast Surg 2016;32:22–8.

36. Hamilton GS. Nasal tip surgery. In: Thomas JR, editor. Advanced therapy in facial plastic and reconstructive surgery. 1st edition. Shelton (CT): People's Medical Publishing House/Enterprise Drive; 2010. p. 800.

37. Sinno S, Chang JB, Saadeh PB, et al. Anatomy and surgical treatment of the depressor septi nasi muscle. Plast Reconstr Surg 2015;135(5):838e–48e.

38. Bewick JC, Buchanan MA, Frosh AC. Internal nasal valve incompetence is effectively treated using batten graft functional rhinoplasty. Int J Otolaryngol 2013;2013(1):1–5.

39. Apaydin F. Nasal valve surgery. Facial Plast Surg 2011;27(2):179–91.

40. Ballert J, Park S. Functional rhinoplasty: treatment of the dysfunctional nasal sidewall. Facial Plast Surg 2006;22(1):049–54.

41. Ghosh A, Friedman O. Surgical treatment of nasal obstruction in rhinoplasty. Clin Plast Surg 2016; 43(1):29–40.

42. Hamra ST. Repositioning the lateral alar crus. Plast Reconstr Surg 1993;92(7):1244–53.

43. Lee M, Guyuron B. Dynamics of the subdomal graft. Plast Reconstr Surg 2016;137(6):940e–5e.

44. Barham HP, Knisely A, Christensen J, et al. Costal cartilage lateral crural strut graft vs cephalic crural turn-in for correction of external valve dysfunction. JAMA Facial Plast Surg 2015;17(5):340.

45. Motamedi KK, Stephan SJ, Ries WR. Innovations in nasal valve surgery. Curr Opin Otolaryngol Head Neck Surg 2016;24(1):31–6.

46. Teichgraeber JF, Gruber RP, Tanna N. Surgical management of nasal airway obstruction. Clin Plast Surg 2016;43(1):41–6.

47. Guyuron B, Bigdeli Y, Sajjadian A. Dynamics of the alar rim graft. Plast Reconstr Surg 2015;135(4): 981–6.

48. Lawson W, Reino AJ. Reduction columelloplasty. A new method in the management of the nasal base. Arch Otolaryngol Head Neck Surg 1995;121(10): 1086–8.

49. Menger DJ. Lateral crus pull-up: a method for collapse of the external nasal valve. Arch Facial Plast Surg 2006;8(5):333–7.

50. Paniello R. Nasal valve suspension: an effective treatment for nasal valve collapse. Arch Otolaryngol Head Neck Surg 1996;122(12):1342–6.

51. White JR, Hamilton GS. Mitek suspension of the lateral nasal wall. Facial Plast Surg 2016;32:70–5.

52. Rhee JS, Book DT, Burzynski M, et al. Quality of life assessment in nasal airway obstruction. Laryngoscope 2003;113(7):1118–22.

53. Rhee JS, Poetker DM, Smith TL, et al. Nasal valve surgery improves disease-specific quality of life. Laryngoscope 2005;115(3):437–40.

54. Chambers KJ, Horstkotte KA, Shanley K, et al. Evaluation of improvement in nasal obstruction following nasal valve correction in patients with a history of failed septoplasty. JAMA Facial Plast Surg 2015; 17(5):347.

55. Chung V, Lee AS, Scott AR. Pediatric nasal valve surgery: short-term outcomes and complications. Int J Pediatr Otorhinolaryngol 2014;78(10): 1605–10.

56. Chung YS, Seol J-H, Choi J-M, et al. How to resolve the caudal septal deviation? Clinical outcomes after septoplasty with bony batten grafting. Laryngoscope 2013;124(8):1771–6.

57. Palesy T, Pratt E, Mrad N, et al. Airflow and patient-perceived improvement following rhinoplastic correction of external nasal valve dysfunction. JAMA Facial Plast Surg 2015;17(2):131.

58. Silva Filho Rde O, Pochat VD. Anatomical study of the lateral crural strut graft in rhinoplasty and its clinical application. Aesthet Surg J 2016;36(8): 877–83.

59. Constantian MB, Clardy BR. The relative importance of septal and nasal valvular surgery in correcting airway obstruction in primary and secondary rhinoplasty. Plast Reconstr Surg 1996;98(1):38–54.

Functional Rhinoplasty

Oren Friedman, MD[a],*, Erdinc Cekic, MD[b], Ceren Gunel, MD[c]

KEYWORDS

• Nasal anatomy • Nasal function • Nasal physiology • Functional rhinoplasty

KEY POINTS

- Understanding nasal anatomy and physiology are the most important points for successful functional rhinoplasty.
- Anatomic structures playing major roles in nasal breathing functions include the septum, and internal and external nasal valves, so physical examination of these regions is essential.
- Planning for functional rhinoplasty involves the identification of the sites of nasal airway obstruction or old trauma, and addressing those regions during the operation with a number of different techniques that have been described.

INTRODUCTION

The nose is the most prominent sensory organ of the face and has 2 important functions: breathing and olfaction. Air passes through the nose, where it is filtered, humidified, and warmed. The nasal organ creates and transmits air of ideal quality into the lungs for optimal gas exchange. To serve this sophisticated function, the nose is composed of an intricate intranasal anatomy and physiologic functionality. As surgeons, we are able to change only the anatomic structures of the nose, thereby increasing airflow, but we are unable to alter nasal physiology.

Rhinoplasty is a surgical procedure that changes both the internal and external shape of the nose. Patients who express a desire for specific changes to the nasal shape, for example, reducing a dorsal hump, changing the shape of the nasal tip, straightening a crooked nose, narrowing the bridge or tip, are seeking elective "cosmetic or aesthetic rhinoplasty." To distinguish, the "functional rhinoplasty" patient seeks improvements in nasal breathing and olfaction, without changes to the shape of the nose. In most cases, functional improvements may be achieved without significantly altering the shape of the nose, such as when we perform septoplasty

and certain types of nasal vestibular stenosis (valve) repair. Many patients want to maintain the existing shape of the nose, and our challenge in these situations is to create improved function and widening of the internal airway while maintaining their existing unique external nasal shape. "Reconstructive rhinoplasty" for congenital or acquired deformities requires changes to the shape of the nose externally to restore or improve the nasal shape or functions; these reconstructive functional rhinoplasties that restore the nose to its premorbid condition should not be considered an elective cosmetic operation. Examples of these situations include cleft lip nasal deformity, old traumatic nasal deformities, and nasal deformities following cancer resection; in these examples, the shape change is aimed at reconstructing the nose or restoring the nose to its premorbid appearance and functional status.

In all types of modern rhinoplasty, even in operations aimed at exclusively cosmetic changes to the nose, it is essential that the surgeon counsel the patient preoperatively that preservation or improvement of breathing is paramount to achieve satisfactory long-term results. The surgeons must themselves understand and then explain to the patient that overaggressive narrowing of the

[a] Clinical Otorhinolaryngology – Head and Neck Surgery, Facial Plastic Surgery, University of Pennsylvania, 3400 Spruce Street, Philadelphia, PA 19104, USA; [b] Otorhinolaryngology – Head and Neck Surgery, Luttiye Nuri Burat State Hospital, 2106 Street No: 8, Sultangazi, Istanbul 34265, Turkey; [c] Otorhinolaryngology – Head and Neck Surgery, Faculty of Medicine, Adnan Menderes University, Kepez Mevkii, Efeler, Aydin 09010, Turkey
* Corresponding author. Penn Medicine, 800 Walnut Street, 8th Floor, Philadelphia, PA 19004.
E-mail address: oren.friedman@uphs.upenn.edu

Facial Plast Surg Clin N Am 25 (2017) 195–199
http://dx.doi.org/10.1016/j.fsc.2016.12.004
1064-7406/17/© 2017 Elsevier Inc. All rights reserved.

nose in the upper, middle, or lower thirds may lead to long-term nasal obstructive symptoms with associated negative quality-of-life implications.[1] Various rates of functional problems after cosmetic rhinoplasty have been reported in the literature, ranging from 15% to 68%,[2–4] and nasal airway obstruction was found to be the most common indication for secondary surgery.[5] Modern rhinoplasty requires that we navigate the patient's desires, and match them with the correct operation, be it purely cosmetic, purely functional with changes made only for breathing, or a combination of aesthetic changes alongside functional breathing improvements.

ASSOCIATION BETWEEN NASAL ANATOMY AND FUNCTION

There are many anatomic structures that contribute to normal nasal function, including the nasal hairs, nostrils, nasal valves, septum, and inferior turbinates. It is commonly believed that internal nasal valve (INV) obstruction, external nasal valve collapse, and septal deviation are the major causes of nasal airway obstruction and are the primary targets in functional rhinoplasty.[6] Understanding and then recognizing the root causes and specific anatomic sites of nasal obstruction in a given patient are keys to successful surgical planning and outcomes.

THE NASAL SEPTUM

The nasal septum is the central structure of the nasal cavity and is formed by the quadrangular cartilage anteriorly, and the perpendicular plate of the ethmoid bone and vomer posteriorly. The septum should lie relatively straight down the nasal midline to support the nose's shape and function.[7,8] The cause of a deviated septum may be traumatic or congenital. "Septal deviations" vary depending on their location (eg, caudal, posterior, anterosuperior) and severity (mild, moderate, or severe). There are also different types of surgical techniques for these different types of deviations. Killian[9] first described the submucous resection technique in 1905, and this technique became increasingly popular over time. In the 1960s, Cottle and colleagues[10] reported a septoplasty technique, and it was accepted as the standard practice for several decades; however, it became clear that correction of the deviated septum by conventional techniques is not always possible. In particular, caudal septal deviations remain a challenge, as manipulation or removal of the caudal septal support risks losing tip support and creating nasal deformities. Traditional

scoring or wedge cartilage excision maneuvers may not be enough in many situations, and it is often important to secure the septum's new midline position to the periosteum of the maxillary crest or nasal spine. In cases of severe deformities of the septum in general, including the caudal and dorsal septum (C-shaped or S-shaped), extracorporeal septoplasty techniques may be used. This technique includes the total or near total removal of the septal cartilage, reshaping and reinforcing a new and strong septal cartilage L-strut, and finally, replacing the removed cartilage into the septal space and fixing it in position. This technique is complicated and time-consuming, and sometimes it becomes hard to reestablish proper nasal support due to deficient cartilage supply. In these cases, costal cartilage or other grafting materials may be used.

THE INFERIOR TURBINATES

The inferior turbinates are lateral nasal wall structures and can easily be seen on anterior rhinoscopy. These structures are composed of bone, a cavernous sinusoid plexus, and an overlying respiratory mucosa. The nasal cycle, autonomic nervous system triggers, and different environmental conditions can alter the cavernous sinusoids so that they may become enlarged due to blood rushing in. Long-lasting, chronic hypertrophy of the inferior turbinates may cause nasal airway obstruction, especially in the nasal valve region where the anterior turbinate head may reduce the nasal valve area. Various surgical methods are described in the literature for turbinate reduction. Turbinate surgery may be considered after failure of topical anti-inflammatory treatments. Lateral out-fracture, submucosal diathermy, electrocautery, and turbinate reduction are the most frequent surgical methods, but we try to avoid the removal of any tissue in most situations. Destruction and excessive removal of respiratory mucosa may cause atrophic rhinitis and subsequent empty nose syndrome. Turbinate surgery is considered only if absolutely necessary, ideally using those techniques that preserve all of the nasal mucosa. Preservation of maximum nasal mucosa allows the nose to best serve its functions of filtration, humidification, and warming.

The popularity of turbinate surgery has been noted to decrease after our understanding of the valve region has become more widespread.[11] Patients very often obtain satisfactory functional benefits from correction of nasal valve and septal deformities without turbinate resection surgery. Turbinates may be crushed and repositioned rather than resected.

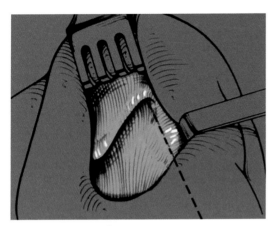

Fig. 1. Illustration of an INV.

INTERNAL NASAL VALVE

The INV area (**Fig. 1**) is bordered by the caudal septum, caudal aspect of upper lateral cartilages (ULCs), head of the inferior turbinate, and the remaining tissues of the surrounding pyriform aperture.[12] The INV is the narrowest portion of the nasal passage and therefore creates the greatest resistance to airflow. The internal nasal valve angle should normally measure between 10° and 20°, and efforts to improve breathing at the level of the INV generally do so through widening of this angle.[13]

There are numerous causes of INV compromise, including congenital sidewall flaccidity, aging, and trauma. Previous nasal surgery involving over-resection of the dorsal hump and division of the ULCs from the septum without reconstructing the attachment are the most common reasons for constriction of the INV area. Incisional intra-nasal scars can also cause stenosis of the INV.[14]

The middle vault, or the nasal valve area, is the most critical region for nasal breathing. The relationship between the ULCs and the septum may be altered from birth, aging, trauma, or from prior rhinoplasty causing middle third narrowing.[15] Spreader grafts (**Figs. 2** and **3**) are often used to reconstruct the middle vault. Placement of spreader grafts under an intact connection between the ULCs and the septum can significantly widen the INV angle better than after division of the ULCs from the septum, together with hump resection.[16] Autospreader flaps, using the upper lateral cartilages to act as spreader grafts, are a nice alternative to middle vault reconstruction with septal cartilage spreader grafts.[17]

Another technique to reconstruct the middle vault is described by Guyuron and colleagues[16] as a splay graft. The graft is harvested from conchal cartilage and is placed on the undersurface of the ULCs and over the dorsum of the septum to reconstruct the middle vault.

The butterfly graft (**Fig. 4**) is highly effective in correcting INV obstruction. It widens the INV angle by flaring the ULCs. Conchal cartilage is harvested, then the graft is carved and secured to the superficial surface of the native upper lateral cartilage with a single stitch on each side. The butterfly graft can be placed through an endonasal or external approach. The dorsal septum can be slightly reduced to create space for the graft to help avoid polly-beak deformity. One of the concerns with the butterfly graft is the negative cosmetic changes that can occur with the application of a cartilage onlay graft along the dorsum and sidewalls of the nose. With practice, the graft may be placed in a way that creates relatively little cosmetic widening of middle third, and relatively little ridge along the dorsum of the nose. However, the proper patient who is selected for this outstanding functional rhinoplasty approach must be willing to accept the possibility of a wider nose as the price for outstanding nasal breathing, otherwise it is not the ideal operation selection.[18]

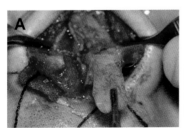 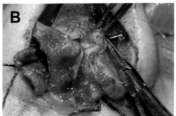 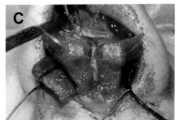

Fig. 2. Dorsal onlay spreader grafts. First described by Craig Murakami[26], these grafts are carved to lay on the nasal bridge, and may often be used to raise the dorsal height if necessary. The onlay graft rests on the dorsal septum and is then secured to the upper lateral cartilage on either side of the nose with suture. Most often, 5 to 0 polydioxanone suture is used. The graft widens the middle third of the nose and thereby increases the nasal valve area and nasal airway. The clinical photos demonstrate the application of the dorsal onlay graft (A), and the suturing of the graft to the upper lateral cartilage (B, C).

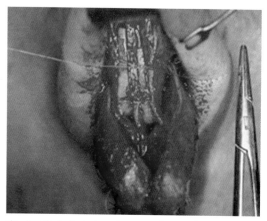

Fig. 3. Clinical photo of a spreader graft.

Various suture techniques have been described to expand the INV angle. The nasal valve flaring suture, a horizontal mattress suture between the ULCs on either side of the nose, have the purpose of widening the INV angle.[19] There also exists a suture technique for the suspension of the cephalic border of the lower lateral cartilages to the lower border of the orbital maxillary periosteum.[20]

EXTERNAL NASAL VALVE

The external nasal valve (ENV) is the region surrounded by the caudal septum and the lateral and medial crura of the lower lateral cartilages. The external valve is located caudal to the INV. Obstruction at either the internal or external valve regions can be static, meaning that the magnitude of obstruction is not affected by negative inspiratory forces created by respiration. In contrast, dynamic collapse of the sidewall is triggered by the inspiratory negative pressures that are generated, and that obstruct nasal breathing on inspiration.[14] Factors that predispose toward collapse of the

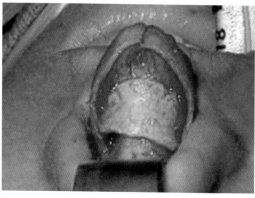

Fig. 4. Clinical photo of a butterfly graft.

ENV include congenital anomalies, trauma, previous surgery, aging, narrow pyriform aperture, and nasal tip ptosis.[21,22] In many revision cases, the lateral crura of the lower lateral cartilages is weakened due to over-resection of the lower lateral cartilages during rhinoplasty, thereby weakening ENV support.

Various cartilage grafts may be used to strengthen ENV stability. The most common technique is the alar batten graft, which may support the weakest points along the nasal sidewall or the alar rim. Alar batten grafts and lateral crural strut grafts provide support and strength to the lateral nasal walls to prevent static and dynamic collapse. These grafts may be placed via an intercartilaginous, marginal, or external incision, including the alar-facial stab approach. Septal, auricular, or rib cartilage graft materials may be used. Depending on where the points of greatest collapse exist, that will determine the location of graft placement. For alar rim graft repair of the external valve, a marginal incision is made and a precise pocket is created in the direction of the alar-facial groove. In the alar-facial stab approach, an incision is made in the alar-facial crease, then blunt dissection through the fibro fatty tissue of the ala is performed to create a pocket into which a cartilage graft is placed.[23,24] Alar rim grafts may help to reinforce the alar rim in cases of cephalic malposition of the lower lateral cartilage, thereby providing a functional solution to lower-third nasal deficiencies without significantly changing the shape of the nose, making it a very simple, quick, effective, and appropriate technique in functional rhinoplasty.[15] When incorporating osteotomies in functional rhinoplasty, as might occur when operating on a patient who presents many years after a traumatic injury, care must be taken to prevent the development of postosteotomy nasal obstruction. To avoid overly narrowing the nasal vault and causing functional breathing problems after osteotomy, Webster and colleagues[25] described the high-low-high osteotomies.

SUMMARY

Understanding nasal anatomy and physiology are the most important points for successful functional rhinoplasty. Anatomic structures playing major roles in nasal breathing functions include the septum, INV, and ENV, so physical examination of these regions is essential. Planning for functional rhinoplasty involves the identification of the sites of nasal airway obstruction or old trauma, and addressing those regions during the operation with a number of different techniques that have been described.

REFERENCES

1. Rhee JS, Poetker DM, Smith TL, et al. Nasal valve surgery improves disease-specific quality of life. Laryngoscope 2005;115(3):437–40.
2. Foda HM. Rhinoplasty for the multiply revised nose. Am J Otolaryngol 2005;26(1):28–34.
3. Chauhan N, Alexander AJ, Sepehr A, et al. Patient complaints with primary versus revision rhinoplasty: analysis and practice implications. Aesthetic Surg J 2011;31(7):775–80.
4. Yu K, Kim A, Pearlman SJ. Functional and aesthetic concerns of patients seeking revision rhinoplasty. Arch Facial Plast Surg 2010;12(5):291–7.
5. Thomson C, Mendelsohn MJ. Reducing the incidence of revision rhinoplasty. Otolaryngology 2007;36(2):130–4.
6. Constantian MB, Clardy RB. The relative importance of septal and nasal valvular surgery in correcting airway obstruction in primary and secondary rhinoplasty. Plast Reconstr Surg 1996;98:38–58.
7. Tardy ME, Thomas JR, Roeder J, et al. Reconstructive surgery of the deviated septum and nose. Washington, DC: Richards Manufacturing Co. Inc; 1982. p. 1–19.
8. Nolst Trenite GJ. Concepts in septorhinoplasty: rhinoplasty, a practical guide to functional and aesthetic surgery of the nose. Part III, chapter 25, 3rd edition. Amsterdam: Kugler Publications; 2004.
9. Killian G. The submucosus window resection of the nasal septum. Ann Otorhinolaryng 1905;14:363.
10. Cottle MH, Loring RM, Fischer GG, et al. The maxillapremaxilla approach to extensive nasal septum surgery. AMA Arch Otolaryngol 1958;68(3):301–13.
11. Afifi AM, Kempton SJ, Gordon CR. Evaluating current functional airway surgery during rhinoplasty: a survey of the American Society of Plastic Surgeons. Aesthetic Plast Surg 2015;39(2):181–90.
12. Apaydin F. Nasal valve surgery. Facial Plast Surg 2011;27:179–91.
13. Goudakos JK, Fishman JM, Patel K. A systematic review of the surgical techniques for the treatment of internal nasal valve collapse: where do we stand? Clin Otolaryngol 2016;42(1):60–70.
14. Motamedi KK, Stephan SJ, Ries WR. Innovations in nasal valve surgery. Curr Opin Otolaryngol Head Neck Surg 2016;24:31–6.
15. Ghosh A, Friedman O. Surgical treatment of nasal obstruction in rhinoplasty. Clin Plast Surg 2016;43:29–40.
16. Guyuron B, Michelow BJ, Englebardt C. Upper lateral splay graft. Plast Reconstr Surg 1998;102:2169–77.
17. Yoo S, Most SP. Nasal airway preservation using the autospreader technique: analysis of outcomes using a disease-specific quality-of-life instrument. Arch Facial Plast Surg 2011;13:231–3.
18. Friedman O, Coblens O. The conchal cartilage butterfly graft. Facial Plast Surg 2016;32:42–8.
19. Schlosser RJ, Park SS. Surgery for the dysfunctional nasal valve. Cadaveric analysis and clinical outcomes. Arch Facial Plast Surg 1999;1:105–10.
20. Paniello RC. Nasal valve suspension. An effective treatment for nasal valve collapse. Arch Otolaryngol Head Neck Surg 1996;122:1342–6.
21. Friedman O, Koch CA, Smith WR. Functional support of the nasal tip. Facial Plast Surg 2012;28:225–30.
22. Kridel RW, Konior RJ. Controlled nasal tip rotation via the lateral crural overlay technique. Arch Otolaryngol Head Neck Surg 1991;117:411–5.
23. Deroee AF, Younes AA, Friedman O. External nasal valve collapse repair: the limited alar-facial stab approach. Laryngoscope 2011;121:474–9.
24. Kovacevic M, Wurm J. Cranial tip suture in nasal tip contouring. Facial Plast Surg 2014;30:681–7.
25. Webster RC, Davidson TM, Smith RC. Curved lateral osteotomy for airway protection in rhinoplasty. Arch Otolaryngol 1977;103(8):454–8.
26. Murakami C. Nasal valve collapse. Ear Nose Throat J 2004;83(3):163–4.

Osteotomies Demystified

Kyle K. VanKoevering, MD[a], Andrew J. Rosko, MD[a],
Jeffrey S. Moyer, MD[a,b,*]

KEYWORDS

- Functional rhinoplasty • Osteotomy • Percutaneous • Crooked nose • Dorsal hump
- Wide nasal dorsum

KEY POINTS

- A methodical preoperative evaluation is critical to understanding the cosmetic and functional concerns of the patient when planning for nasal osteotomies.
- An inconsistent variety of osteotomy nomenclature is used for osteotomy classification. However, the key concept of picture framing the nasomaxillary complex is critical to reproducible results.
- Perforating percutaneous osteotomies are gaining in popularity owing to the ease of access and reduction in postoperative edema and ecchymosis.

The osseous framework of the nose provides the structural foundation for both nasal shape and function. The paired nasal bones join the ascending (or frontal) process of the maxilla, defining the upper lateral sidewall and dorsal width in conjunction with the upper lateral cartilages. Superiorly, the nasal bones join the nasal part of the frontal bone, defining the nasion. Superolaterally, the frontal process of the maxilla joins the frontal bone, completing the bony nasal vault.[1] These osseous structures are concealed by the overlying skin, soft tissue, and nasal mimetic musculature within the superficial musculoaponeurotic system.[2] Alterations in the shape and orientation of the bony framework may be congenital or acquired in nature (ie, posttraumatic). However, these alterations can have significant cosmetic and functional impacts that can be concerning to the patient.

The approach to the surgical management of the bony nasal vault remains challenging and is frequently debated among rhinoplasty surgeons.[1–5] As the osseous framework provides the foundation from which the remainder of the structural elements of the external nose are derived, operative management is complex and nuanced. To improve management and outcomes, it is imperative to follow a comprehensive and structured preoperative evaluation.

EVALUATION OF THE BONY NASAL VAULT

Evaluation of the nasal framework starts with a comprehensive history. It is important to elicit the specific functional and/or cosmetic complaints of the patient. Use of a hand-held mirror can be beneficial as the patient describes their primary concerns. Prior history of trauma or past nasal surgery could suggest increased scar formation and adhesions, potential fracture lines, and possibly less structural tissue integrity in comparison with congenital cases. Past medical history is also important, because a history of autoimmune diseases affecting the nose, chronic steroid use, or cardiopulmonary disease among other findings may all affect the operative and anesthetic approach.

After eliciting a comprehensive history, a systematic physical examination is performed.

Disclosure Statement: The authors have nothing to disclose.
[a] Division of Facial Plastic and Reconstructive Surgery, Department of Otolaryngology – Head and Neck Surgery, University of Michigan, 1500 East Medical Center Drive, 1904 Taubman Center, Ann Arbor, MI 48109-5312, USA; [b] Center for Facial Cosmetic Surgery, 19900 Haggerty Road, Suite 103, Livonia, MI 48152, USA
* Division of Facial Plastic and Reconstructive Surgery, Department of Otolaryngology – Head and Neck Surgery, University of Michigan, 1500 East Medical Center Drive, 1904 Taubman Center, Ann Arbor, MI 48109-5312.
E-mail address: JMoyer@med.umich.edu

Structurally, the nose can be divided horizontally into the osseous, cartilaginous, and lobular thirds roughly corresponding with the nasal bones, upper lateral cartilages, and lower lateral cartilages, respectively.[6] Focusing on the upper third, evaluation should be performed from both the frontal and the lateral views. Palpation is critical to evaluate for bony step-offs, instability, and the thickness of nasal skin overlying the nasal bones. From a frontal view, nasal bone abnormalities can be categorized into deviations and width abnormalities of the vault.[3] The nasal bones should project symmetrically along the sagittal midline. Prior trauma or congenital abnormalities can project the nasal root off the midline. When evaluating the bony width of the nose, the dorsal and ventral width must be evaluated. The dorsal width is defined by the nasal bones at the dorsal projection, helping to contour the brow–tip aesthetic line, while the ventral width is defined by the ascending process of the maxilla.[7] Cochran and colleagues[7] describe that the ventral width should be about 80% of the alar width in the ideal nose; however, this can vary based on gender and race. Notice should be made of a narrow dorsum, particularly as a result of prior osteotomies that may be causing functional obstruction. From the lateral view, one should evaluate the nasofrontal angle and the radix height. Classically, the ideal nasofrontal angle for the Caucasian male ranges from 115° to 130°, although this, too, can vary significantly based on gender and race.[8,9] Again from the lateral view, evaluation for a dorsal hump is critical, because this is often a prominent cosmetic concern. The need to address a dorsal hump operatively is a key consideration in planning for potential osteotomies. The details of the nasal anatomy must be taken in the context of the facial profile, including forehead profile, dental occlusion, and chin projection.[10]

Preoperative photography is an excellent, objective means to document findings regarding the bony nasal vault and to plan approaches for operative repair. Traditional facial plastic photography should be used, including the anteroposterior, oblique, and lateral views.[11] Ideally, this should be performed in a photo studio with a lighting system to avoid shadows, and with reference to the horizontal Frankfort line.[12] These photographs allow the surgeon to frame the discussion with the patient, and help to illustrate concerns that may be encountered. The photographs should be taken to the operating room to provide a reference for the operative plan.

The decision to proceed with rhinoplasty including osteotomies is a complex decision that requires a detailed understanding of the nasal anatomy and a comprehensive evaluation. Generally speaking, osteotomies are best suited for correction of a deviated dorsum, thinning of a broad nasal dorsum, or closing open roof deformities. Rarely, osteotomies can be used to widen an excessively thin dorsum from previous surgery.[13] This review aims to highlight the critical considerations and components in nasal osteotomies.

PERIOPERATIVE CONSIDERATIONS

Planning for rhinoplasty procedures in which osteotomies may be indicated is imperative. In addition to patient photography and a detailed discussion regarding desired outcomes, an appropriate anesthetic and operative setup are critical to success.

Anesthesia

Rhinoplasty procedures are performed under a wide array of anesthetic plans, including local anesthesia, sedation with local anesthetic, and general anesthesia. The choice of anesthesia is also related to overall patient comorbidities. For relatively straightforward soft tissue rhinoplasty procedures, some advocate for the use of local anesthetic and sedation over general anesthesia, citing less bleeding and postoperative pain.[14,15] Sklar and colleagues[15] describe performing approximately 80% of their rhinoplasty cases under local with sedation rather than general anesthesia, even when performing routine osteotomies and dorsal hump rasping. However, when cases are expected to take longer than 80 minutes, involve relatively complex structural reshaping, or patients who are not American Society of Anesthesiologists class I or II, they typically prefer general anesthesia. Although definitive data may be lacking, a systematic review and metaanalysis on the management of nasal bone fractures showed that general anesthesia was favored over local anesthesia (with or without sedation) for closed reduction of nasal bone fractures. The metaanalysis showed that trends for patient satisfaction with anesthesia, nasal function, and need for subsequent anesthesia all favored general anesthesia and there was a statistically significant improvement in cosmetic satisfaction when patients underwent general anesthesia.[16] These data suggest that cosmetic outcomes when manipulating the bony vault could be improved under general anesthesia, but the data are far from definitive and the decision should be made on a case-by-case basis.

Adjunct Medications

A handful of adjunct medications have been studied in rhinoplasty to reduce bleeding or postoperative effects. Tuncel and colleagues[17] found that the use of controlled hypotension intraoperatively with perioperative steroids significantly reduced intraoperative bleeding as well as postoperative edema and ecchymosis. Notably, a regimen of 3 doses of dexamethasone (at the start of the operation, at the time of the osteotomy, and 24 hours postoperatively) resulted in statistically less edema at postoperative days 5 and 7 compared with a single dose. A subsequent meta-analysis similarly demonstrated both edema and ecchymosis in rhinoplasty patients was significantly improved with perioperative steroids and that multiple steroid doses seemed to be superior.[18] Ong and colleagues[19] recently published a similar systematic review confirming the usefulness of steroids, as well as intraoperative hypotension, cooling, and postoperative head elevation in reducing postoperative complications. We routinely use perioperative steroids in rhinoplasty cases, as well as perioperative cooling and head elevation, particularly when osteotomies are planned.

More recently, the usefulness of desmopressin for hemostasis in rhinoplasty, particularly with osteotomies, has been described. Initially described in orthognathic surgery,[20] Gruber and colleagues[2,21] have more recently published on the benefits in nasal osteotomies. They recommend IV dosing of 0.1 μg/kg, typically giving a maximum of 3 doses intraoperatively to assist with bleeding and ecchymosis. Although data are sparse, there have been no reported thrombotic complications and it may offer hemostatic benefits beyond traditional local epinephrine.[1,15]

OPERATIVE TECHNIQUES

Although the indications and desired outcomes from nasal osteotomy are well-established, the nomenclature, approach, and technique for these osteotomies remains clouded with considerable confusion and debate. In general, an osteotomy is defined as a controlled fracture or cut in the bony pyramid of the nose. Traditionally, this has been performed with a "continuous" osteotomy— a controlled, continuous curvilinear cut (classically performed with a saw or osteotome) completely transecting the bone.[5,22] More recently, "perforating" osteotomies have gained momentum. Perforating osteotomies are performed as a postage-stamp style of discrete, discontinuous small osteotomies (typically 2-3 mm) along the desired fracture line.[23] The bone is then manually fractured along this line in a controlled fashion, theoretically reducing the soft tissue trauma and subsequent ecchymosis and edema. In an effort to standardize the nomenclature around osteotomies, we have classified osteotomies into 4 types: medial, lateral, transverse, and intermediate. The various approaches, techniques, and limited data supporting them are discussed for each.

The general principle of nasal osteotomies is to mobilize each nasomaxillary complex. This includes the nasal bone and a segment of the ascending process of the maxilla. It is important to note that lateral osteotomies are placed through the maxilla, rather than the nasal bone. This concept involves "picture framing" the bony dorsum to completely mobilize each half. The senior author generally approaches complete mobilization through a medial and lateral osteotomy, which is connected by a transverse osteotomy for full mobilization.

Medial Osteotomy

As the name suggests, the medial osteotomy is performed medially along the nasal bone, separating it from the septum and contralateral nasal bone. In general, this osteotomy is aligned primarily along the parasagittal plane, although a wide array of oblique angles and variations are described.[1,2] Notably, much of the dissection and manipulation of the medial osteotomy is aided by digital palpation because visualization is limited with the open or endonasal approach.

Dorsal hump

A discussion regarding medial osteotomies should include dorsal hump reduction. In a significant portion of patients undergoing osteotomies, the reduction of the dorsal hump is often a key component in the reshaping of the osseous nasal vault. A dorsal hump is a prominence at or near the rhinion and can be bony and/or cartilaginous.[24] There are multiple techniques described for managing a hump. Joseph and Skoog initially described the use of an osteotome to remove the medial nasal bones along with the dorsal septum and medial upper lateral cartilages.[25] Given the inherent limitations in visualization, this en bloc technique can result in overresection or asymmetry. Therefore, conservative reduction is critical. Once the dorsal hump is excised, an open roof deformity is created. Careful planning must be performed before the bony cut in the dorsal nasal bones is performed. Detailed marking of the skin and the subsequent osteotomy trajectory can be beneficial in avoiding asymmetry. The brow–tip aesthetic lines follow along the contour of the dorsal bony width. This line, along with the projection of the nose from lateral view, can assist the surgeon in planning.

An alternative to the osteotome and en bloc excision of the dorsal nasal bones, many surgeons use a rasp to sequentially file the bony hump.[10,26,27] With this approach, the cartilaginous portion is managed sharply. However, the bony dorsum is reduced with either a pull or push rasp. The key advantage of the rasp is the slower, controlled reduction of the bony hump. Frequent redraping of the soft tissue envelope allows the surgeon to gauge the degree of hump reduction that has been performed and evaluate for symmetry.

With either approach, complete removal of the dorsal hump simultaneously completes the medial osteotomy as the nasal bones are mobilized from the septum. Some authors promote extending an obliquely angled medial osteotomy from the hump reduction[2]; however, this is typically not necessary if combined with a complete lateral and transverse osteotomy, because the transverse osteotomy serves the same function.[10]

The final point of discussion regarding hump reduction is the importance of an open roof deformity. After excising the dorsal hump, the dorsum is left with a flat and wide contour as the nasal bones are separated from the septum. This contour irregularity is referred to as an "open roof" deformity, and results in a prominent dorsal width if not corrected. Correction requires mobilization of the nasomaxillary bone complex and infracture to reduce the width.

Traditional medial osteotomy

If a dorsal hump reduction is not performed, a traditional medial osteotomy is typically required to separate the nasal bones from the septum. A wide array of medial osteotomy trajectories have been described, including fading, straight, and oblique variations.[1] Gruber and colleagues described a wedge of thick, hypervascular bone along the medial, cephalad nasal bones. We prefer to avoid this bone with a gently fading medial osteotomy technique. With this technique, the osteotome is engaged in the caudal edge of the nasal bone adjacent to the septum. The osteotome is initially angled vertically then slowly directed approximately 15° lateral to the sagittal plane (**Fig. 1**A).[28] It is important to note that the medial osteotomy primarily controls the dorsal width. The final consideration in the medial osteotomy is the length of the cut. As the osteotome is gently faded off the sagittal plane, it is imperative to complete the osteotomy before reaching the nasofrontal suture. If the osteotomy is extended through the nasofrontal suture, the thick cephalic bone fulcrums or "rocks" about the suture, resulting in lateralization of the cephalic segment with medialization of the caudal nasal bone. This complication,

referred to as a rocker deformity, can be readily visualized through the thin dorsal skin. It can be corrected by performing a transverse osteotomy caudal to the nasofrontal suture line and the nasal bone can then be manipulated without fulcruming across the suture.

Lateral Osteotomy

As the name suggests, the lateral osteotomy is performed laterally to mobilize the nasal framework. Notably, the lateral osteotomy is performed through the ascending process of the maxilla and not the nasal bone.[1] This is critical to avoid an obvious bony stepoff within the nasal contour.[3] The lateral osteotomy is fundamental in mobilizing the nasal bones and allowing for closure of an open roof deformity. The location of the osteotomy also determines the ventral width of the bony dorsum. In general, this osteotomy is arranged in a more coronal or mixed sagittal–coronal orientation and is a critical tool in the shaping of the osseous dorsum (**Fig. 1**B). However, the orientation of the lateral osteotomy and subsequent infracture can significantly influence the cross-sectional area of the internal nasal valve and nasal airway.[4] Despite these key concepts, there continues to be considerable debate surrounding the best methods for performing the lateral osteotomy. More so than with medial osteotomies, the described approaches for the lateral osteotomy have been highly variable, including endonasal, sublabial, and percutaneous approaches with perforating and continuous osteotomies.[1,29,30] Similarly, an even greater and more confusing array of orientations and trajectories have been described, including "high–high," "low–low," "low–high," "high–low," and "high–low–high" among others.[1,2,10,29] These orientations will be addressed in more detail below.

Endonasal approach

Traditionally, the lateral osteotomy is performed via endonasal access.[10] First, the planned osteotomy trajectory is marked cutaneously. A small stab incision is made in the nasal mucosa at the level of the pyriform aperture (the starting location depends on the desired trajectory). This should be started just above the level of the inferior turbinate attachment. A small amount of bone at the pyriform aperture should be preserved to prevent overnarrowing of the nasal airway. A gentle dissection is carried through the incision to the lateral surface of the maxilla.[1,2] Some surgeons prefer to elevate the periosteum off the nasal process of the maxilla along the tract of the proposed osteotomy. The usefulness of periosteal elevation remains a topic of debate; in theory, elevating the periosteum protects it from the osteotome and helps to hide bony

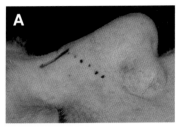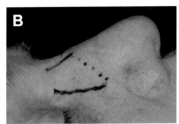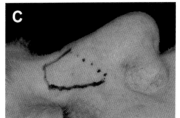

Fig. 1. Picture framing of the nasomaxillary complex using a gently fading medial osteotomy (*A*), paired with a standard lateral osteotomy up to the level of the medial canthus (*B*), and joined with a transverse osteotomy (*C*). The dotted line represents the caudal edge of the osseous vault.

stepoffs. However, a recent systematic review demonstrates increased postoperative ecchymosis with periosteal elevation.[19] In either case, a guarded osteotome is then guided along the proposed trajectory of the planned lateral osteotomy by manual palpation in a continuous fashion toward the medial canthus. Some authors advocate for a similar endonasal approach combined with a perforating lateral osteotomy, which avoids a skin incision but requires skilled manipulation of the osteotome along the perforated osteotomy course.[1]

Percutaneous approach

More recently, a percutaneous approach to the lateral osteotomy has been advocated. Initially popularized in the 1990s, the percutaneous approach uses a small cutaneous stab incision, typically at the midpoint of the planned osteotomy.[23,31] Typically, a 2-mm straight osteotome is then inserted through the incision down to the nasal process of the maxilla (**Fig. 2**A).[1] Using detailed palpation and following the marked path of the planned osteotomy, a series of small, discrete osteotomies are performed along the trajectory with shallow punches through the bone. Palpation is key to effectively "postage stamp" the cut,

leaving 1- to 2-mm segments of intact bone between each osteotomy without disrupting the underlying nasal mucosa, preserving stability to the nasal bones.[4] There is no periosteal dissection performed, and the postage stamp leaves strips of periosteum intact along the osteotomy line. The osteotomy is then completed with digital manipulation. This approach has become the preferred approach for lateral osteotomies by the senior author.

In addition to the endonasal and percutaneous approaches, other approaches to the lateral osteotomy have been described. This includes the sublabial approach as described by Ghassemi and colleagues,[30] which is particularly beneficial for so-called low access to the pyriform aperture, and the transpalpebral approach.[32] Recently, access for the lateral osteotomy was described through wide dissection of the skin and soft tissue envelope laterally over the pyriform aperture.[33] Using the traditional "open sky" approach, the authors claimed to have sufficient access to the pyriform without complication. However, each of these approaches involve increased soft tissue dissection with significant postoperative ecchymosis and edema from the extended dissection. In general, these alternative approaches are

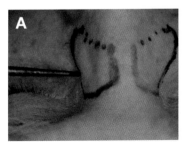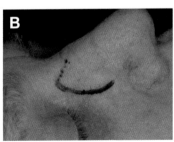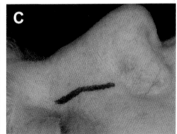

Fig. 2. Variations of lateral osteotomy techniques. Percutaneous approach (*A*) typically performed with a 2-mm, straight, unguarded osteotome through a small incision in the lateral nasal wall, postage-stamping a perforated osteotomy along the marked trajectory. One could also use a "low–high" lateral osteotomy paired with a medial oblique osteotomy (*B*). The medial oblique osteotomy is often paired with an open roof, performing the same function as the transverse osteotomy. A "low–low" osteotomy trajectory (*C*) can also be used to narrow the ventral width more aggressively.

reserved for unique clinical situations and have limited data supporting improved efficacy.

Lateral osteotomy trajectories

As noted, the literature is scattered with various "paths" for the lateral osteotomy. These trajectories include "high" and "low" descriptions with regard to the anatomic position from lateral view of the nose. Thus, a "high" location is more anteromedial in the osseous vault, and a "low" trajectory is more posterolateral. Reliably and accurately performing the planned osteotomy is critical to the success of the procedure. The osteotomy is generally finished anterior to the medial canthus and caudal to the frontomaxillary suture. Many advocate for starting the osteotomy "high" in the vault just cephalad to the head of the inferior turbinate (the so-called Webster's triangle) to avoid infracturing of the turbinate and narrowing of the airway.[10,22] However, others support a lower starting position inferolaterally in the pyriform aperture to more efficiently mobilize the ventral base (**Fig. 2**B,C).[2] Controversies such as this over the best trajectory have failed to demonstrate a clearly superior approach. This is likely because each patient should have an individualized approach based on the ventral width, facial profile, intercanthal distance, ethnic, gender background, nasal airway, and desired outcome. An osteotomy that is taken too "high" may fail to correct the broad ventral width and leave a palpable bony stepoff, whereas an osteotomy taken to "low" into the maxilla may injure the nasolacrimal duct or narrow the nasal airway significantly with infracture.

Another key concept is asymmetric osteotomies when correcting a deviated dorsum. For example, when the bony pyramid is deviated to the right, the right nasomaxillary complex is shorter, and the left nasomaxillary complex is flatter but longer. The lateral osteotomy on the right would need to be made "lower" or more posterolaterally than the left to allow the dorsum to remain level once mobilized to the left. A critical understanding of the nasal anatomy is imperative to effectively performing these osteotomies, and experience with a variety of osteotomy trajectories can improve the surgeon's repertoire of skills.

Comparative data

There are relatively limited data comparing osteotomy techniques. Perhaps most studied has been a comparison of the perforating (internal or external) versus continuous osteotomy approach. Gryskiewicz and Gryskiewicz[34] found that a percutaneous perforating lateral osteotomy resulted in reduced postoperative ecchymosis and edema when compared with continuous osteotomy in a prospective, randomized study, and has been confirmed in subsequent evaluations.[35] The percutaneous approach may result in visible scarring postoperatively, although the incidence has been reported to be quite low (3%–6%).[36,37] Zoumalan and colleagues[38] found there is no difference in the ability of perforating versus continuous osteotomies in successfully reducing the ventral width. Collectively, these data suggest that the perforating osteotomy is reliable and equally successful, compared with the continuous osteotomy, in mobilizing the ventral osseous structures and may result in less nasal trauma and fewer postoperative sequelae.

Instrumentation

The final point of consideration in the lateral osteotomy is the instrument of choice. Traditional osteotomes come in a variety of sizes and shapes, including single and double guarded osteotomes, curved, and notched. Many have suggested thinner osteotomes (3 mm or less) are beneficial in reducing surrounding soft tissue trauma.[3,34] Curved osteotomes can be beneficial for nonlinear continuous cuts. Osteotome sharpness was evaluated by Bloom and colleagues[39] and demonstrated that osteotomes dull quickly and that professional resharpening may provide only modest benefits. More recently, the usefulness of piezoelectric instruments has been evaluated and found beneficial in making controlled osteotomies while minimizing soft tissue trauma.[40–42] The frequencies used for bone cuts are different than those used for soft tissue and authors suggest minimal trauma. However, direct comparison with conventional osteotomes has not been performed.

Transverse Osteotomy

The concept of picture framing the bony nasal structure with osteotomies is critical to controlled and precise nasal reshaping. Complete mobilization requires not only a medial and lateral osteotomy, but also an osteotomy that joins these 2 cuts to allow for complete, controlled mobilization. Alternatively, greenstick fracturing between the 2 osteotomies can be performed, but is uncontrolled. The nomenclature about this portion of nasal osteotomies has been inconsistent. Some authors describe a laterally angulated component of the medial osteotomy to approach the end of the lateral osteotomy. This has a wide variety of names, including the lateralized medial oblique osteotomy, fading, or medial oblique osteotomy.[2,5,10,43] Yet others describe a "high" lateral osteotomy at the cephalic margin that sweeps medially as it approaches the frontal bone toward the medial osteotomy.[1,7,29] We prefer a separate, distinct "transverse" osteotomy that joins the medial and lateral osteotomies in the nasal root, caudal to the nasofrontal suture. Thus, we distinctly discuss the transverse osteotomy as a separate osteotomy that completes the picture framing of the nasomaxillary complex (**Fig. 1C**).

The transverse osteotomy is oriented in a more axial plane. Transverse osteotomies can be performed as continuous osteotomies, as in the medial oblique osteotomy (**Fig. 2B**), or more commonly as percutaneous osteotomies, particularly when placed more cephalad, limiting direct exposure.[2,7] In the percutaneous approach, a similar, small transverse stab incision can be performed midway along the course of the transverse osteotomy. The transverse osteotomy is postage stamped in a similar fashion. Once completed and the entire nasal framework has been osteotomized, digital infracture or outfracture with a Boies elevator completely mobilizes the bony segment along the defined osteotomy tract. One important consideration is the concept of an asymmetric transverse osteotomy for correcting the deviated dorsum. By way of example, if the dorsum is deviated to the right, the transverse osteotomies should be performed more obliquely such that each osteotomy trajectory moves more inferiorly as it travels from right to left. This allows the nasomaxillary complexes to be infractured and outfractured respectively, ending at the same height.

Modifications to the transverse osteotomy have been described. Avsar[44] more recently described the use of an oscillating saw for performing transverse osteotomy via an endonasal approach, assisted with an endoscope. The en block osteotomy for the severely deviated dorsum has also been described. This procedure involves a transverse osteotomy across the entire nasal root, connecting paired lateral osteotomies without a medial osteotomy. This process allows for the entire bony pyramid to be mobilized en block.[3] In the absence of medial osteotomies, connection to the nasal septum must be divided. This undertaking is useful only in the most severe deviations in which dorsal hump removal (and thus medial osteotomies) are not used.

Given the low rate of perceivable scarring and more direct access with the percutaneous approaches, this has become the standard practice for many surgeons. Whether viewed as a distinct osteotomy or incorporated into the medial or lateral osteotomy, the transverse portion of picture framing of the bony pyramid is a critical component to controlled mobilization of the nasomaxillary complex (**Fig. 3A, C**).

Intermediate Osteotomy

The final osteotomy type is the intermediate osteotomy. The intermediate osteotomy is performed relatively parallel to the medial osteotomy, but

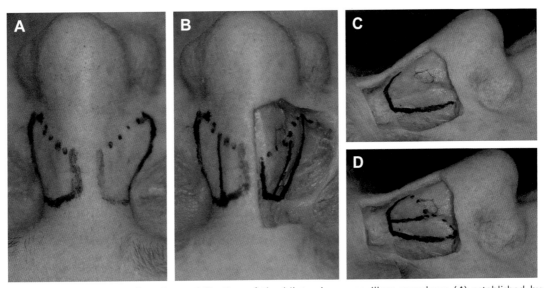

Fig. 3. Paired osteotomy plans for mobilization of the bilateral nasomaxillary complexes (*A*) established by palpating the bony landmarks. Having removed the skin and soft tissue envelope over the right dorsum, the planned osteotomies are retraced, now including an intermediate osteotomy (*B*). Lateral profile of medial, lateral, and transverse osteotomy trajectories after removal of skin and soft tissue envelope (*C*) and addition of planned intermediate osteotomy (*D*) at the nasomaxillary suture. Dotted line represents the caudal edge of the osseous vault.

positioned more laterally in the nasal bone. The concept is to divide the nasomaxillary bony complex into 2 distinct segments: roughly the nasal bone and the ascending process of the maxilla (**Fig. 3**B, D). This is particularly beneficial in patients with a wide dorsal width and convex nasal bones. The convex shape of the nasal bones prevents the surgeon from being able to adequately narrow the dorsum unless the nasomaxillary complex is reoriented into a more concave shape.[10] This allows for a smoother transition to the dorsum closure and is more aesthetically pleasing. The concept could also be applied to severely concave nasal bones.[1] The intermediate osteotomy allows the bony pyramid to be rearranged in multiple segments, allowing for even greater mobility. In addition to the correction of a convex nasal bone, it can also be used to "comminute" the nasomaxillary complex for straightening of the severely deviated dorsum, and may often be used unilaterally to correct significant asymmetry. However, with increased mobility comes increased risk for delayed healing and visible or palpable step-offs as a result of malunion. Access to the intermediate osteotomy is typically via traditional open approach like the medial osteotomy, though this can also be performed percutaneously.[10] The osteotome is engaged at the caudal end of the lateral nasal bone and the osteotome is directed superiorly to intersect the transverse osteotomy near the junction with the medial osteotomy. The sequence of osteotomies is particularly important, especially when performing an intermediate osteotomy. If the entire nasomaxillary complex has been mobilized by the picture framing osteotomies (medial, lateral, and transverse), it is nearly impossible to complete the intermediate osteotomy on the mobile fragment.[1] Thus, we recommend performing this osteotomy before the lateral osteotomy is performed. In the senior author's hands, the intermediate osteotomy is relatively uncommon in practice, but a critical tool for the severely deviated or convex nasal bone.

Postoperative Care

Although it is clear the osteotomies increase postoperative edema and ecchymosis, the use of steroids and cooling have proven beneficial.[18,19] Nasal packing was shown to increase edema and ecchymosis postoperatively and should be used judiciously.[19] An external splint is used routinely in our practice after nasal osteotomy, and is generally a standard practice. Varedi and Bohluli[45] demonstrated a trimmed external splint may function better than a larger splint at helping the nasal bones to maintain shape. We generally keep the splint in place for 1 to 2 weeks postoperatively. According to the American Association of Plastic Surgeons recent consensus statements, antibiotic prophylaxis is recommended for rhinoplasty and is our standard practice.[46] Typically, these antibiotics are prescribed for 7 days postoperatively.

SUMMARY

Nasal osteotomies are critical components in shaping the nasal dorsum. The primary indications are closing an open roof deformity (from hump removal), narrowing a broad dorsum, widening an overly thinned dorsum, or straightening a deviated dorsum. There are a wide variety of approaches, trajectories, and tools used in performing nasal osteotomies, and a standardized classification such as the one proposed could help to simplify the literature. Preoperative considerations are critical in planning the proper osteotomies and understanding a patient's desired outcome is imperative to success. Perforating osteotomies are gaining in popularity because they seem to be equally reliable to traditional continuous osteotomies while resulting in fewer postoperative complications. There continues to be debate over the proper approach to each of these osteotomy patterns, but understanding the patient's specific anatomy should allow the surgeon to perform a wide variety of approaches to accomplish the desired results. This strategy is important for maintaining the nasal airway and avoiding complications. The concept of picture framing of the nasomaxillary bone to be mobilized is critical to predictable fracture patterns and reproducible results. In our experience, this is best accomplished with medial, lateral, and transverse osteotomies. Intermediate osteotomies are used less frequently, but provide more mobility to reshape highly convex or severely deviated nasal bones. Postoperative care is critical to the long-term success of the rhinoplasty. With a detailed understanding and a thorough approach to nasal osteotomies, the contour and function of the bony vault can be successfully reshaped for a successful outcome for both the surgeon and patient.

REFERENCES

1. Bloom JD, Immerman SB, Constantinides M. Osteotomies in the crooked nose. Facial Plast Surg 2011; 27(5):456–66.
2. Gruber RP, Garza RM, Cho GJ. Nasal bone osteotomies with nonpowered tools. Clin Plast Surg 2016; 43(1):73–83.
3. Wayne I. Osteotomies in rhinoplasty surgery. Curr Opin Otolaryngol Head Neck Surg 2013; 21(4):379–83.

4. Ozucer B, Ozturan O. Current updates in nasal bone reshaping. Curr Opin Otolaryngol Head Neck Surg 2016;24(4):309–15.

5. Most SP, Murakami CS. A modern approach to nasal osteotomies. Facial Plast Surg Clin North Am 2005; 13(1):85–92.

6. Palhazi P, Daniel RK, Kosins AM. The osseocartilaginous vault of the nose: anatomy and surgical observations. Aesthet Surg J 2015;35(3):242–51.

7. Cochran CS, Ducic Y, Defatta RJ. Rethinking nasal osteotomies: an anatomic approach. Laryngoscope 2007;117(4):662–7.

8. Leong SC, White PS. A comparison of aesthetic proportions between the healthy Caucasian nose and the aesthetic ideal. J Plast Reconstr Aesthet Surg 2006;59(3):248–52.

9. Leong SC, White PS. A comparison of aesthetic proportions between the Oriental and Caucasian nose. Clin Otolaryngol Allied Sci 2004;29(6):672–6.

10. Azizzadeh B, Reilly M. Dorsal hump reduction and osteotomies. Clin Plast Surg 2016;43(1):47–58.

11. Swamy RS, Most SP. Pre- and postoperative portrait photography: standardized photos for various procedures. Facial Plast Surg Clin North Am 2010; 18(2):245–52. Table of Contents.

12. Swamy RS, Sykes JM, Most SP. Principles of photography in rhinoplasty for the digital photographer. Clin Plast Surg 2010;37(2):213–21.

13. Angelos PC, Been MJ, Toriumi DM. Contemporary review of rhinoplasty. Arch Facial Plast Surg 2012; 14(4):238–47.

14. Dogan R, Erbek S, Gonencer HH, et al. Comparison of local anaesthesia with dexmedetomidine sedation and general anaesthesia during septoplasty. Eur J Anaesthesiol 2010;27(11):960–4.

15. Sklar M, Golant J, Solomon P. Rhinoplasty with intravenous and local anesthesia. Clin Plast Surg 2013; 40(4):627–9.

16. Al-Moraissi EA, Ellis E 3rd. Local versus general anesthesia for the management of nasal bone fractures: a systematic review and meta-analysis. J Oral Maxillofac Surg 2015;73(4):606–15.

17. Tuncel U, Turan A, Bayraktar MA, et al. Efficacy of dexamethasone with controlled hypotension on intraoperative bleeding, postoperative oedema and ecchymosis in rhinoplasty. J Craniomaxillofac Surg 2013;41(2):124–8.

18. Hwang SH, Lee JH, Kim BG, et al. The efficacy of steroids for edema and ecchymosis after rhinoplasty: a meta-analysis. Laryngoscope 2015;125(1):92–8.

19. Ong AA, Farhood Z, Kyle AR, et al. Interventions to decrease postoperative edema and ecchymosis after Rhinoplasty: a systematic review of the literature. Plast Reconstr Surg 2016;137(5):1448–62.

20. Guyuron B, Vaughan C, Schlecter B. The role of DDAVP (desmopressin) in orthognathic surgery. Ann Plast Surg 1996;37(5):516–9.

21. Gruber RP, Zeidler KR, Berkowitz RL. Desmopressin as a hemostatic agent to provide a dry intraoperative field in rhinoplasty. Plast Reconstr Surg 2015; 135(5):1337–40.

22. Webster RC, Davidson TM, Smith RC. Curved lateral osteotomy for airway protection in rhinoplasty. Arch Otolaryngol 1977;103(8):454–8.

23. Goldfarb M, Gallups JM, Gerwin JM. Perforating osteotomies in rhinoplasty. Arch Otolaryngol Head Neck Surg 1993;119(6):624–7.

24. Arslan E, Aksoy A. Upper lateral cartilage-sparing component dorsal hump reduction in primary rhinoplasty. Laryngoscope 2007;117(6):990–6.

25. Skoog T. A method of hump reduction in rhinoplasty. A technique for preservation of the nasal roof. Arch Otolaryngol 1966;83(3):283–7.

26. Park SS. Fundamental principles in aesthetic rhinoplasty. Clin Exp Otorhinolaryngol 2011;4(2):55–66.

27. Sykes JM, Tapias V, Kim JE. Management of the nasal dorsum. Facial Plast Surg 2011;27(2):192–202.

28. Harshbarger RJ, Sullivan PK. The optimal medial osteotomy: a study of nasal bone thickness and fracture patterns. Plast Reconstr Surg 2001;108(7): 2114–9 [discussion: 2120–1].

29. Bohluli B, Moharamnejad N, Bayat M. Dorsal hump surgery and lateral osteotomy. Oral Maxillofac Surg Clin North Am 2012;24(1):75–86.

30. Ghassemi A, Riediger D, Holzle F, et al. The intraoral approach to lateral osteotomy: the role of a diamond burr. Aesthetic Plast Surg 2013;37(1):135–8.

31. Rohrich RJ, Krueger JK, Adams WP Jr, et al. Achieving consistency in the lateral nasal osteotomy during rhinoplasty: an external perforated technique. Plast Reconstr Surg 2001;108(7):2122–30 [discussion: 2131–2].

32. Amar RE. Correction of the bony rings during the aesthetic rhinoplasty: apologia of the transpalpebral osteotomy. Aesthetic Plast Surg 1998;22(1):29–37.

33. Tellioglu AT, Sari E, Ozakpinar HR, et al. Intranasal extramucosal access: a new access for lateral osteotomy in open rhinoplasty. J Craniofac Surg 2016;27(3):e257–9.

34. Gryskiewicz JM, Gryskiewicz KM. Nasal osteotomies: a clinical comparison of the perforating methods versus the continuous technique. Plast Reconstr Surg 2004;113(5):1445–56 [discussion: 1457–8].

35. Rohrich RJ, Minoli JJ, Adams WP, et al. The lateral nasal osteotomy in rhinoplasty: an anatomic endoscopic comparison of the external versus the internal approach. Plast Reconstr Surg 1997;99(5): 1309–12 [discussion: 1313].

36. Gryskiewicz JM. Visible scars from percutaneous osteotomies. Plast Reconstr Surg 2005;116(6): 1771–5.

37. Hinton AE, Hung T, Daya H, et al. Visibility of puncture sites after external osteotomy in rhinoplastic surgery. Arch Facial Plast Surg 2003;5(5):408–11.

38. Zoumalan RA, Shah AR, Constantinides M. Quantitative comparison between microperforating osteotomies and continuous lateral osteotomies in rhinoplasty. Arch Facial Plast Surg 2010;12(2):92–6.

39. Bloom JD, Ransom ER, Antunes MB, et al. Quantifying the sharpness of osteotomes for dorsal hump reduction. Arch Facial Plast Surg 2011;13(2): 103–8.

40. Robiony M, Toro C, Costa F, et al. Piezosurgery: a new method for osteotomies in rhinoplasty. J Craniofac Surg 2007;18(5):1098–100.

41. Tirelli G, Tofanelli M, Bullo F, et al. External osteotomy in rhinoplasty: piezosurgery vs osteotome. Am J Otolaryngol 2015;36(5):666–71.

42. Pribitkin EA, Lavasani LS, Shindle C, et al. Sonic rhinoplasty: sculpting the nasal dorsum with the ultrasonic bone aspirator. Laryngoscope 2010; 120(8):1504–7.

43. Ghanaatpisheh M, Sajjadian A, Daniel RK. Superior rhinoplasty outcomes with precise nasal osteotomy: an individualized approach for maintaining function and achieving aesthetic goals. Aesthet Surg J 2015;35(1):28–39.

44. Avsar Y. The oscillating micro-saw: a safe and pliable instrument for transverse osteotomy in rhinoplasty. Aesthet Surg J 2012;32(6):700–8.

45. Varedi P, Bohluli B. Do the size and extension of the external nasal splint have an effect on the osteotomy, brow lines, and long-term results of Rhinoplasty: a prospective randomized controlled trial of 2 methods. J Oral Maxillofac Surg 2015;73(9):1843.e1-9.

46. Ariyan S, Martin J, Lal A, et al. Antibiotic prophylaxis for preventing surgical-site infection in plastic surgery: an evidence-based consensus conference statement from the American Association of Plastic Surgeons. Plast Reconstr Surg 2015;135(6):1723–39.

Management of Pediatric Nasal Surgery (Rhinoplasty)

Matthew D. Johnson, MD

KEYWORDS

• Rhinoplasty • Septoplasty • Turbinate • Nasal surgery • Pediatric • Neonatal • Nasal growth

KEY POINTS

- Nasal surgery in children, most often performed after trauma, can be performed safely in selected patients with articulate, deliberate, and conscientious operative plan.
- In addition to form and function, nasal growth is also a consideration.
- Nasal septal abscess and hematoma can lead to long-term changes that benefit from early reconstruction.
- Primary cleft rhinoplasty can improve nasal appearance and reduce severity of cleft-related nasal deformity.
- Neonatal septal deviation may correct itself when minor; severe obstruction can benefit from intervention.

INTRODUCTION

Nasal surgery in the pediatric patient continues to be controversial. Contention persists on what impact there is to the growing nose.[1] Currently, most surgeons wait until after puberty for elective nasal surgery. Surgery of the nose in children intends to improve function and appearance while preserving conditions for future development and growth. There are potential effects of misdirected growth after trauma in which significant deviation is exacerbated during nasal growth. Likewise, it remains unclear what the effect of surgical intervention is on growth. The current state of thought holds that surgery of the nose and septum should be avoided in prepubescent children, unless severe derangement, trauma, mass, or congenital defect exist to avoid risk of growth center disruption.

Rhinoplasty in children has been met with mixed opinions. Initially, it was thought that surgery should be avoided at all costs when it pertained to a child's nose. Over time, after investigation, this thinking changed. It is now believed that well-thought-out and deliberate surgery of the child's nose can improve the nasal airway and the nasal aesthetics and even optimize growth.

HISTORICAL PERSPECTIVE

First descriptions of pediatric rhinoplasty date back to 1902.[2] The next decade followed with reports of adverse effects: saddle nose, growth inhibition, and maxillary retrusion.[3] After early sequelae of nasal surgery were identified, there was a movement for avoidance of all surgery on the child's nose. Between the 1950s and the 1970s literature warned about disrupting the septal cartilage owing to its role in ventral and caudal projection[4] or resecting the keystone area before completion of growth.[4,5] The sentiment was to delay surgery until growth was complete believing severe disturbance would interfere with further development.[5]

Facial Plastic & Reconstructive Surgery, Division of Otolaryngology - Head and Neck Surgery, Southern Illinois University School of Medicine, 747 N Rutledge Street, 5th floor, PO box 19649, Springfield, IL 62794-9649, USA
E-mail address: mjohnson81@siumed.edu

Facial Plast Surg Clin N Am 25 (2017) 211–221
http://dx.doi.org/10.1016/j.fsc.2016.12.006

ANIMAL STUDIES

Animal studies were performed in the 1950s and 1960s on various models. The most prominent were completed by Sarnat and Wexler[6,7] using a rabbit model resecting septal cartilage with perichondrium, which resulted in dramatic impairment of nasal and midface growth. Hartshorn[8] showed altered growth in canines repeating the study. Squier and colleagues[9] examined histology showing that fibrosis after resection may contribute to a pattern of restricted growth. However, study in Guinea pigs with varied amount of resected cartilage only showed variable growth when extensive cartilage was resected.[10] Fuchs[11] showed impacted growth with only resecting perichondrium. Bernstein,[12] in a canine model, preserved the mucoperichondrium, elevating flaps and removing septal cartilage or autotransplanting cartilage. Autografted septum remained viable and removed areas had regeneration of cartilage at 10 months. Additional study of maneuvers consistent with septorhinoplasty and perichondrial preservation in ferrets showed no change to facial growth on cephalogram[13]

NASAL ANATOMY AND GROWTH
Embryology

The region within the frontonasal process differentiates into nasal placodes, which invaginate to a pit, eventually becoming the nasal passages and choana. Each nasal pit is flanked by part of the lateral and medial nasal prominence. In the midline, the medial nasal prominences fuse, ultimately becoming central nasal structures and the philtrum. The maxilla, arising from the first arch, the maxillary prominence, moves medially with the lateral nasal process to fuse with the combined medial nasal prominence. These processes are complete at around 10 weeks. During fifth to seventh week of gestation, ossification centers arise for maxilla and nasal bones. By the eighth week, vomer ossifies. Chondrification of lateral nasal walls happens during the third month. At the sixth month, cartilages differentiate from a single unit into upper lateral cartilage (ULC), lower lateral cartilage (LLC), and septal cartilage.[4]

Anatomy

There are distinct differences in the child's nose compared with the adult nose, beginning with smaller dimensions. Even during childhood, the amount of cartilage and the profile of the nose changes. The overlying skin and soft tissue contains more fat and is generally thicker than that in the adult nose. The T-bar complex forms much of the nasal support.[14] The pediatric nose has typical differences from that of the adult. The septum has variable thickness. The tip is slightly elevated and less projected with an increased nasolabial angle. The tip is flat and the columella is short. The dorsal length is reduced. The nares are small and rounded.[14–16] The nasal vestibule is smaller in children comparatively, which can limit exposure in endonasal surgery.[17]

Septum

The septum in an infant's nose has significantly more cartilage than bone compared with that of an adult. In the infant, septal cartilage spans from the nasal spine to the sphenoid rostrum.[18,19] There are thicker areas corresponding to growth centers and thinner areas that are at risk for fracture during injury.[14]

Perpendicular plate and vomer

Vomer arises from progressive ossifying fragments flanking a basal of cartilage along the palatal bone.[14] Endochondral ossification adjacent to the skull base in ventrocaudal direction results in the perpendicular plate. Nasal growth proceeds with both continued ossification and cartilage growth. By age 6 to 8 years, the perpendicular plate and vomer reach contact with each other.[1]

Lateral cartilages

The ULC extends superiority under the nasal bones.[14,18,19] The dorsoseptal T bar, composed of septum and upper lateral cartilages, fused initially, is the main support in neonates and children.

Nasal bones

Nasal bones are shorter. The suture lines remain open. As in adults, they include the nasal process of frontal bones and ascending process of the maxilla completing the bony nasal vault.

Growth

There are 2 periods of nasal growth: the first occurs during the initial 2 to 5 years of life, the second is during puberty.[15] The septal cartilage in children is similar in size to adult cartilaginous septum by 2 years of age. There is continued enlargement in the dorsocaudal direction and enlargement of the bony proportion of septum.[20] The pubertal nasal growth occurs between ages 12 and 16 years for girls and 15 and 18 years for boys. Additional studies found continued increases in nasal growth to age 20 in women and 25 in men.[21] The nasal septum has been shown to grow until age 36 years.[20]

Nasal septal cartilage is thought to be a driving factor in nasal growth (**Fig. 1**). During fetal development, as the cartilaginous structures are fusing, the sphenoid rostrum grows anteriorly meeting the posterior septum. The vomer develops bilaterally, posteriorly, and inferiorly to the cartilage septum. It fuses and ossifies as it grows forward.[14] The suture line between the vomer and premaxilla is an important growth center. This suture line is abnormal in orofacial clefts and may contribute to the observed asymmetric growth disturbances. Septal cartilage growth centers include the sphenospinal and sphenodorsal regions. Nasal bones develop over the triangular cartilage capsule, absorbing this precursor of the bony pyramid.[14] As the LLC extends downward, the tip becomes more bulbous and drops, and the nares are no longer visible. The LLC becomes more resilient and firms in adolescence. Nasal dorsal height and anterior-posterior projection increase.[14]

Abnormal Growth

Septal deviation present during the rapid phase of development can cause irregular growth and amplify the deviation. Compelled oral breathing, such as in severe obstruction, disrupts normal craniofacial and maxillofacial growth.[22] Altered craniofacial development, similar that of adenoid facies, from open mouth, anterior tongue placement, and decreased maxilla facial tone, changes the developmental forces. Septal deviation produces a pattern of narrow maxilla, maxillary protrusion, arched palate, malocclusion, micrognathia, retrognathia, and an increased anterior lower vertical facial height.[23–26]

Cartilage Regeneration

In children, after cartilage injury, the response may be loss, incomplete regeneration, or complete regeneration. In adults, regeneration is not observed; rather, fibrosis in child and adult cartilaginous fractures never heal, they fibrose between segments. Histologically, regenerated cartilage seems to have random arrangement of chondrocytes.[27] Intact perichondrium is necessary to facilitate regeneration. Excessive regeneration can be detrimental causing undirected growth, even to the point of new obstruction.[27]

NASAL DEFORMITIES

Nasal deformity in children primarily arises from trauma or inheritance. Both of these contribute to early and late deformities. Nasal masses and congenital malformations are additional causes. Intrauterine growth restriction, birth injury, and familial characteristics can all lead to preadolescent deformity.

Nasal abnormality can be classified by the timing of when it was thought to have occurred (ie, prenatal, neonatal, infant). Perhaps more useful is classifying by contributing forces: trauma, trauma with growth, growth alone, or developmental. The last category includes congenital anomalies.

PATIENT EVALUATION

Nasal airway obstruction (NAO) is a common finding in the pediatric population; the variety of etiologies includes adenoid hypertrophy, septal deviation, turbinate hypertrophy, nasal polyposis, and nasal tumors. NAO in children often has multiple causes, rarely owing solely to septal deviation.[17] Symptoms include: diminished quality of life, chronic rhinitis, mouth breathing, sleep-disordered breathing (SDB), and obstructive sleep apnea (OSA). Associated symptoms include recurrent sinusitis, malocclusion, and recurrent otitis media.[28] Uncorrected septal deformities worsen over time and can impact frequency of these symptoms.[29]

An appropriate and thorough evaluation identifying the contributing factors may find ways to avoid need for surgery.[17] The examination should include anterior rhinoscopy to assess degree of septal deflection/deformity and flexible fiberoptic

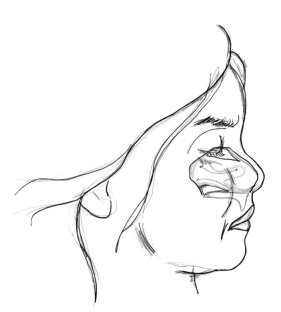

Fig. 1. Septal growth centers: thickened septal cartilage present in the sphenospinal and sphenodorsal areas. The anterior region contains thinner cartilage.

examination to aid in finding the pathology of NAO and eliminating others. It is prudent to perform endoscopy in pediatric patients before surgery. Computed tomography is rarely needed unless there is concern for a mass or posterior anomaly.[30]

NASAL SURGERY

All pediatric nasal surgery has the goals of improving the nasal airway, restoring normal anatomy and appearance, and preservation of growth potential. These goals are accomplished by conservative surgery with restoration of the nasal framework, projection, dorsum, tip, and tip position.[31] There remains no consensus to absolute or relative indications for surgery. Generally accepted indications for surgery include septal hematoma or abscess, severe deformity from acute trauma, reconstruction after removal of nasal mass, and cleft lip nasal deformity. Severely deviated septum causing significant NAO or anticipated progressive distortion of the nose with growth is considered by many a reasonable indication for intervention.[17] Procedure selection should consider the patient's anatomy and goals of surgery. An external approach would be best in cases of free graft technique or septal explant with autologous grafting.[31]

TURBINATES

Turbinate hypertrophy is a common cause of pediatric NAO. In the past, turbinate surgery was performed via multiple methods. Resection of partial or complete turbinate was favored in the early 1990s, followed in late 1990s with transition to the use of lasers. Currently, submucosal microdebridement and radiofrequency thermal ablation are favored.[32-34]

Typically, children are treated medically for 3 months before considering surgery for turbinates. Hypertrophy can be bony or mucosal. Examination of the turbinates should include response to topical decongestants. Surgery is offered empirically, depending on reported symptoms and clinical assessment.[35] A recent survey study of practice patterns in pediatric turbinate surgery reported indications for surgery of 82% for nasal obstruction and 16% for SDB.[36] It was the only procedure 20% of the time and concomitant with others in 80%, typically with adenotonsillectomy, septoplasty, or sinus surgery.[36] The overall complication rate is around 4%,[35] with the most common complication being intranasal synechiae. Others include epistaxis, pain, or nasal crusting. There are no reports of atrophic rhinitis.

Sullivan and colleagues[34] found improved respiratory parameters in pediatric patients who underwent adenotonsillectomy with inferior turbinate reduction versus those who underwent adenotonsillectomy alone. Improvement in sleep parameters was documented on polysomnography. A review by Leong and colleagues[35] reported Oxford Centre for Evidence-Based Medicine grade C recommendation to support inferior turbinate reduction in children. No studies have long-term follow-up results, as such long-term efficacy and impact on facial growth, if any, is unclear. The natural history of turbinate hypertrophy in children also lacks data. Severe turbinate hypertrophy contacting the septum is hypothesized to cause septal deviation. Despite poor evidence and lack of long-term outcomes, it is still a reasonable treatment in children with medically nonresponsive chronic rhinitis, OSA/SDB, NAO, and mild-to-moderate septal deviation to avoid nasal surgery.

SEPTOPLASTY

Septal surgery is reasonable after age 5 to 6 years when performed appropriately.[37] Avoiding surgery in children with severely deviated nasal septum (DNS) can lead to facial abnormalities, malocclusion, and respiratory symptoms.[38,39] Endonasal approaches are typically used, such as Killian or hemitransfixion incisions. Visualization can be difficult, especially in very young patients. A sublabial approach can improve access. Endoscopic assistance can aid in seeing and targeting areas. Often spurs can be removed by elevation of an ipsilateral submucoperichondrial flap. A microdebrider can be used to precisely remove a spur or specific area of deviation.[17] With broad deviations, the convex surface of the cartilage can be scored to relax the deviation. Deviated cartilage can be resected and reimplanted.[39] Excess cartilage can be judiciously excised. With any repair, superimposing segments of cartilage or bone should be avoided. Christophel and Gross[17] highlight pitfalls and techniques to optimize operations on the nasal septum. They emphasize the fragile nature of mucoperichondrium, clearly important to preserve for cartilage survival and thus growth. An endoscope can be instrumental in visualization. And whenever possible, bone and cartilage should be restored to its position after straightening.[17]

- Preserve perichondrium
- Preserve cartilage, avoid large resections, no submucosal resection
- Maintain the bony-cartilaginous junction whenever possible
- Remodel and reposition cartilage

RHINOPLASTY

Pediatric rhinoplasty generally is defined as rhinoplasty in girls less than 14 and boy less than 16 years of age. Selecting appropriate patients (trauma, tumor, congenital anomaly) with preservation of key structures and sparing use of grafts will provide benefit.[1] Rhinoplasy is most commonly used in cases of deformity and dysfunction after nasal trauma and severe crooked nose accompanied by functional impairment. It may also be considered in severe deformity, after tumor resection, and for cleft nasal deformity or other congenital reasons.[1] The argument for surgical intervention includes redirection of what would have been abnormal and deviated growth as well as the benefits of improved nasal airway function, aesthetics, and positive psychosocial impacts.

To a degree, the goals of surgery will vary according to the etiology: after trauma, return to pre-injury state; after tumor or mass removal, restoring premorbid nasal function; in congenital malformations, creating a more normal anatomic configuration. As above, conservation of septal structures is key. As in adults, ensuring adequate septum for tip support is important. Cautious grafting is paramount, since even though the proportion of cartilaginous septum is higher, less cartilage is available for graft creation.[30] Grafting is used when required to ensure tip projection, position, and support. Auricular cartilage and small amounts of septum are available. Maintaining the T-bar of ULC and septum keeps the dorsum stable. In removal of dorsal structures or with total septal reconstruction, spreaders are necessary to stabilize and sustain midline dorsal support. Spreader grafts can also stabilize a severe dorsal deviation toward the midline.[30] Native structures are preserved when possible, resection is conservative, and improvements are achieved through sculpting, augmentation, and other changes.[30] The objective is not to create the sculpted adult nose but restore function with age-appropriate appearance.[1,30] Medial and lateral osteotomies can be performed to center the nasal pyramid, especially after trauma. Osteotomies can be performed through previous fracture lines.[22] Dorsal hump reduction is best postponed until after puberty. Consideration should be taken of age, severity of associated septal deviation, and further growth potential. When performing the procedure, native length and projection of the nose should be kept.[30] Saddle defects of the dorsum may require grafting to recreate normal nasal dimensions.[30]

- Keep maximal structure allowable while achieving goals
- Minimize grafting
- Maintain caudal tip support
- Consider spreaders for dorsal strength where appropriate
- Consider auricular cartilage for grafting
- Reduce dorsal hump only when accompanied by severe deviation
- Medial and Lateral osteotomies may be used in redirecting upper nose

NASAL TRAUMA

Among nasal fractures, 70% occur in children older than 12 years.[40] Etiology is variable by age and includes sports injury (28%), accidental trauma (21%), interpersonal violence (10%), motor vehicle collision (6%), home injury, birth trauma, or nonaccidental trauma.[40,41] Eighty percent felt that closed reduction was satisfactory in the early postoperative period; however, agreement between provider and family on successful return to premorbid appearance has been reported in as few as one-third of cases,[40] leaving a remainder of persistent posttraumatic deformities.

In the young nose, much of the structure is cartilage, which compresses or flexes and is more likely to buckle from trauma. Higher potential for cartilage displacement or fracture exists. Increased incidence of greenstick fractures, splaying, flattening, and cartilage avulsions also result from their anatomy.[30] For this reason, septal hematoma is also more common than in adults. The nasal bones are much smaller compared with those of the adult. As a result, there is less likely to be nasal bone fracture in the very young nose. The extent of injury is often underappreciated.[42]

In addition to normal external and internal nasal examinations, attention must be paid to alar base position, widening of nasal root, and detailed septal examination. Endoscopy may be useful in delineating extent of injury and inspecting the posterior septum. Fracture of nasal bones may be accompanied by nasoethmoidal or orbital fractures, identified by CT imaging when suspected.[41] Imaging studies are typically not helpful in isolated nasal fractures.

Untreated nasal fractures disrupt growth and culminate into well-described deformities: widened dorsum, widened base, short nasal length, short columella, saddling, and tip ptosis. Associated midface changes include short premaxilla, diminished nasal spine, high palate, and elevated occlusal plane.[14,43] Untreated traumatic changes can lead to soft tissue contracture and distortion, making further reconstruction much more difficult.

Pediatric Nasal Fracture Pattern: Nasal Bones

Pediatric nasal fractures have been described as either lateral or frontal.[44] Lateral fractures may result in infracture of the ipsilateral bone and possibly outfracture of the contra lateral bone. The fracture often occurs at the junction between the ascending maxillary process and nasal bone. Forces striking the nose from the front have potential to propagate injury to structures posterior to the nasal bones, such as the lacrimal system and the nasoethmoid region, and may shift the pyramid posterior superiorly. Unfused midline suture between the nasal bones allows for "open book" fracture, which manifests after a frontal injury causes separation and splaying of the nasal bones in the midline (**Fig. 2**).

Pediatric Nasal Fracture Pattern: Septal Fractures

Two common patterns of septal fracture have been described: vertical septal fracture and C-shaped fracture. The vertical septal fracture extends from the dorsum to the spine in the anterior region. The "C-shaped fracture" has an inferior, horizontal component through the thin area of cartilage in the central septum.[14] It begins in the inferior central region, extends posteriorly and superiority into and through ethmoid plate, then travels along dorsum toward the tip (see **Fig. 2**).

Assessment of the fracture pattern will identify patients appropriate for closed reduction. Reduction of nasal bones or septum may be performed under regional nerve block, monitored sedation, or general anesthesia as deemed appropriate per patient age and tolerance. With closed reduction, placement of internal packing and external splint maximizes stability for healing. Dissolvable packing is preferred in young patients. After edema has settled into the nose, closed reduction may

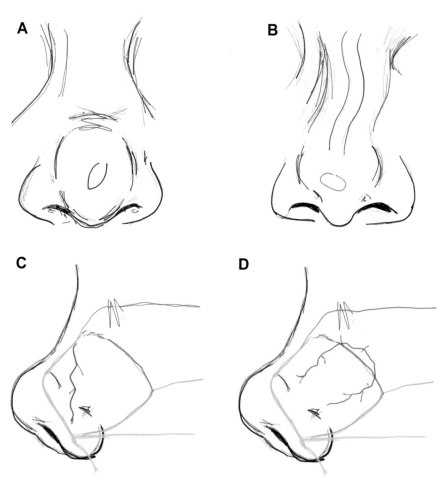

Fig. 2. Nasal bone fractures from a (*A*) frontal injury results in the "open book" or splayed and widened appearance. (*B*) Lateral injury may cause a resulting infracture on the side of injury and outfracture on the opposite side. Septal fracture may be a (*C*) vertical fracture from the dorsum down to the nasal spine region or (*D*) C-shaped deformity through thin regions of septum. Pediatric nasal bone and septal fractures are more prone to shearing of the perichondrium and septal hematoma; the caudal cartilage may be dislocated off the crest, or there may be disarticulation of bony-cartilaginous junction.

need to be delayed for 3 to 5 days or until swelling reduces[41] and is reasonable up to 2 weeks after injury. With both septal and bony displacement, when performing bony reduction, the septal deviation should be addressed; otherwise, recurrence of the injury pattern can result.[45]

An open reduction via septorhinoplasty with or without osteotomies is the next step to reduce a bone or septal injury after failed closed reduction. Generally accepted indications for open surgery are severe septal deviation with NAO, SDB, or OSA. When addressing green stick fracture by open reduction, converting to a full fracture first improves effectiveness of reduction.[17] Fractures that are nonreducible, involve posteroinferior septum, or are located very anterior may require acute open reduction.[41]

Septoplasty can address issues of the quadrangular cartilage that do not involve the dorsal and caudal regions. As in adults, when these areas are involved, a more comprehensive approach is needed in septorhinoplasty. Patient age and degree of skeletal maturity are considered in operative planning. Removing minimal cartilage, preserving ULC-septal relation in the cartilaginous T-bar, and maintaining the bony-cartilaginous junction should be accomplished when possible.[46] Bony deviations can be addressed with precise osteotomies.

NASAL SEPTAL HEMATOMA/ABSCESS

Septal hematoma occurs more often in children after nasal trauma. Septal hematoma can develop from dental or sinonasal infections. In pediatric nasal trauma, 15% of patients may subsequently have nasal septal hematoma.[47] As the cartilage buckles during trauma, submucosal vessels rupture, and without an accompanying tear of mucosa, there is nowhere for the blood to drain. Septal hematoma is treated with incision and drainage followed by compression with septal splints or packing. Left untreated, not only is there high risk of cartilage loss, the hematoma can transition into an abscess. Nasal septal abscess in children is rare, with incidence of 0.9% among pediatric facial trauma.[48] The valveless venous system of the midface poses a risk for retrograde propagation of thrombophlebitis toward the cavernous sinus.[49] Septal abscess is treated similarly with incision-drainage, drain, and intravenous broad-spectrum antibiotics. Microbiology is most often aerobic, predominantly *Staphylococcus aureus*[50,51] mixed with other typical flora of the upper aerodigestive tract. A drain or packing is left in the nose to prevent re-accumulation. Destruction of the nasal septal cartilage is possible with appropriate treatment and more likely with delays or inadequate care. Loss of septum can result in impaired

midfacial development. Some surgeons advocate for drainage by an external approach with immediate nasal septal reconstruction.[52,53] Autologous grafts such as septal, conchal, and costal are favored and include composite septum constructed with fibrin glue.[54] External approach is preferred, as it affords wide access to the septum. Alternatively, reconstruction is delayed until after puberty. Proponents of early reconstruction believe that it corrects the defect, restores function, and prevents significant midface growth issues. Opponents argue that damaged septal cartilage may yet regenerate.[55] In severe deficits of cartilage with significant deformity, most support early reconstruction.

CLEFT LIP NASAL DEFORMITY

Orofacial clefting has associated nasal malformation. There is deficiency of the ipsilateral maxilla, the bony foundation. The alar base is positioned laterally, inferiorly, and posteriorly in contrast to the noncleft side. The lower lateral cartilage is broad and flattened over its course. There is abnormal muscle insertion and therefore pull. The nasal spine and anterior septum are deviated to the noncleft side. As the septum travels posteriorly, it transitions to a deviation toward the cleft side (**Fig. 3**).

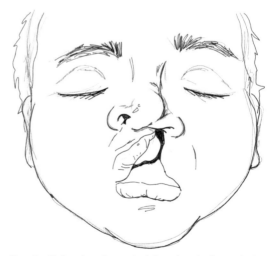

Fig. 3. Cleft-related nasal deformity: ipsilateral alar base displaced laterally and inferiorly. Alar base is posterior secondary to maxillary deficiency. There is fibrofatty tissue thickening the width of the base. The internal nasal lining has attachment to pyriform. The lower lateral cartilage is flattened effacing the dome region. There is an appearance of hooding from inferior displacement of the nasal sil edge. The nasal tip is deviated to the contralateral side and flattened on the ipsilateral side; there may be torsion from ipsilateral columellar shortening. The septum deviates toward the contralateral side anteriorly and to the ipsilateral side posteriorly.

Primary rhinoplasty performed at the time of initial lip repair can diminish the cleft nasal deformity and is becoming the standard of care.[56] Surgical intervention results in scarring, and there have been concerns of impact on future surgery and even growth. Generally, patients with clefting often require definitive septorhinoplasty after puberty. Presurgical nasoalveolar molding is especially useful in wide clefts. The directed constant and changing pressure shapes the nasal soft tissues and can improve position of abnormally placed structures.[57] Lip repair is performed around 3 months of age but maybe later if presurgical nasoalveolar molding is used. Primary rhinoplasty is performed through the lip incisions, which provide access to the columellar base and cleft side alar base. Elevation (supraperichondrial) of the soft tissue off of the LLC, nasal tip, and cleft side ala is done to accomplish redraping. Tip projection is brought toward the midline, improving projection and creating symmetry.[58,59] The cleft side alar base is release from attachments to the pyriform rim allowing for mobilization. It is important to avoid narrowing the nostril at this stage.[58] The nasal vestibule floor is created during lip repair, at a position comparable to the noncleft side. Intranasal and external pledgets sutured into position or internal mattress sutures are used to reposition the LLC. Removing a judicious amount of subcutaneous tissue from the cleft side alar base can reduce excess bulk[58]; pledget placement here compresses the lateral region of the vestibule for shaping. Pledgets/bolsters are removed in 3 to 7 days.[58] Silastic nasal conformers are used for 4 to 6 weeks postoperatively, to improve shape.[60] Goals of primary rhinoplasty include repositioning alar base, creating symmetric arch of LLC, and improving tip position.

Secondary cleft rhinoplasty includes both definitive and intermediate surgeries. Definitive surgery occurs after most nasal growth is complete and the patient is at or near skeletal maturity. Any definitive nasal surgery should be postponed until after planned orthognathic surgery, bone grafting, or anticipated changes in maxilla.[61] Intermediate rhinoplasty may be performed if a lip revision is planned before the start of school (around age 4 to 6 years) or if severe septal deviation is causing significant NAO. A plethora of surgical techniques have been described, and a review is beyond the scope of this article. Intermediate rhinoplasty has similar goals to primary rhinoplasty: improve symmetry with minimal scarring and impact on growth. Definitive rhinoplasty seeks to achieve nasal symmetry and optimal function of the nasal airway.[61]

NEONATAL NASAL AIRWAY OBSTRUCTION

Neonatal patients may be obligate nasal breathers up to 6 months of age. Neonatal nasal airway obstruction has a wide differential diagnosis, including deformity of lateral nasal cartilages, choanal atresia, pyriform aperture stenosis, midnasal stenosis, congenital cysts or masses, abnormal midface growth, or nasal septal deviation. In the neonate with respiratory distress, a thorough workup is warranted, including complete airway, cardiopulmonary, and neurologic systems examination.

Reported rates of neonatal DNS range from 14.5% to 58%, but most studies reported around 15% to 20%.[62] Among these, a smaller proportion has an associated external nasal deformity. An individual's nasal architecture is impacted by familial traits, genetics, race, birth trauma, subsequent trauma, and previous surgery.[62] Neonatal septal deviation falls into 2 categories: anterior displacement off the crest from trauma during birth and a combined (anterior and posterior) deviation resultant from intrauterine forces during fetal growth.[63] Gray[64] suggested that causes of DNS include differential rate of growth compared with other midface structures or nasal trauma from prolonged intrauterine mechanical compression or during parturition. The nose projects from the center of the face and is subjected to multiple forces during the labor and delivery process; thus, microfractures and dislocation occur. In most cases, neonatal septal dislocations return to near normal within a few days. This occurrence seems more likely when the cartilage is bowed but not dislocated or fractured.[65] When persistent and severe, it can mimic symptoms of choanal atresia, complete unilateral obstruction.[62] Features that increase risk of neonatal DNS include increased birth weight, breech position, and vaginal delivery. Incidence is inversely correlated with parity.[62]

Septal deformities that persist beyond the neonatal period can impact the growth and development of the maxilla/midface. Early management, when warranted, has the potential to prevent progression or complications later in life.[62] Owing to its role in midface growth, damage to septal cartilage can lead to significant abnormalities of maxillofacial.[66] Closed septal reduction has been performed within the first 1 to 2 days of life[66] with success in treating anterior subluxations/dislocations of cartilage.

Closed septal reduction has had success, even when performed within 1 to 2 days of life.[67,68] Open septal reduction has been performed via a sublabial approach[69] affording improved visualization. Alternatively, endoscopic-assisted approach through a hemitransfixion incision also provides optimal visualization.[66] Steps are taken to preserve maximal septal cartilage.

LONG-TERM OUTCOMES

Evidence shows that judicious pediatric nasal surgery does not significantly impact nasofacial growth. Nonetheless, it is important to counsel patients about possible influences on growth of the nose. As with trauma, surgery itself can result in altered growth and the possibility that residual or new asymmetries will become apparent over time.

Adil and colleagues[30] highlighted how early literature relating to nasal surgery and growth long term was from transnasal skull base surgery in the pediatric population. Transseptal surgery via sublabial, transseptal, and transsphenoid approaches, performed in children ages 4 years and older, were followed over time. There were no reports of nasal or craniofacial deformity after these procedures. This surgery does not involve resection of septal cartilage but disruption by displacement, for skull base access, and repositioning.

El-Hakim and colleagues[39,70] used anthropometric measures to follow an external approach to septoplasty with autotransplantation compared with age-matched controls and found no change in development of the nose or midface. There was a statistical trend in shortening of the nasal dorsum and tip protrusion.

Dispenza and colleagues[22] looked at long-term results after posttraumatic septoplasty or rhinoplasty in children ages 4 to 12. Outcome was measured by observed deviation of the nose or septum. The follow-up period was 7 to 20 years with only 1 patient having displacement of the inferior portion of the quadrangular cartilage.[22]

Tasca and Compadretti[28] looked at nasal growth after septoplasty via hemitransfixion incision in patients 5 to 12 years of age with follow-up spanning 6 to 14 years. Among their 44 patients, half underwent in situ modifications and the others extracorporeal technique. Results were evaluated by nasal endoscopy and anthropometric nasal measurements. These results were then compared with normative data for age-matched controls. All anthropometric measures were within normal/normative range. With septal explant, there was a trend toward effect on reducing nasofacial angle.[28]

Bejar and colleagues[71] looked at pediatric patients who underwent an external approach to septoplasty with a mean follow-up of 3.4 years. They examined anthropometric measures of nasal and facial growth comparing them with normative data. They observed a trend in shortening of the nasal dorsal length. The remaining measures did not show any deviance from normal growth.

McComb and Coghlan[72] performed primary rhinoplasty at time of cleft lip repair and did not observe any long-term growth effects. They did an 18-year longitudinal study of nasal and midface growth noting no long-term effects. They compared their subjects with age-matched normals and age-matched control subjects with cleft lip who did not have rhinoplasty.[72] They report that symmetry created by nasal surgery persisted into adulthood.

SUMMARY

Understanding of the growing pediatric nose continues to improve. It is possible to perform conscientious nasal surgery in children who have nasal airway obstruction. Each pediatric patient should be evaluated thoroughly with examination and endoscopy. Turbinate surgery can be useful in cases of mild-to-moderate septal deviation to ameliorate symptoms until growth is complete (or a more reasonable time). Closed septal reduction in the neonatal patient may be useful in restoring septal position and may prevent deviated growth. Conservative and limited nasal surgery can be performed in children taking care to preserve maximal amount of septal structure. There may be subtle impacts on growth of the nasal dorsum after more involved surgery. Strong indications for surgery include severe septal deviation, reconstruction after removal of nasal mass, and congenital malformations, such as cleft lip nasal deformity. All nasal surgery in children seeks to avoid disruption of the growth centers, preserving and optimizing nasal growth while improving the form and function of the nose. A solid appreciation of long-term outcomes and effects on growth remain elusive.

REFERENCES

1. Funamura JL, Sykes JM. Pediatric septorhinoplasty. Facial Plast Surg Clin North Am 2014;22:503–8.
2. Freer OT. The correction of deflections of the nasal septum with a minimum of traumatism. JAMA 1902;38:636–42.
3. Hayton CH. An investigation into the results of the submucous resection of the septum in children. J Laryng 1916;31:132–8.
4. Gilbert JG, Segal S Jr. Growth of the nose and the septorhinoplastic problem in youth. AMA Arch Otolaryngol 1958;68(6):673–82.
5. Farrior RT, Connolly ME. Septorhinoplasty in children. Otolaryngol Clin North Am 1970;3(2):345–64.

6. Sarnat BG, Wexler MR. Growth of the face and jaws after resection of the septal cartilage in the rabbit. Am J Anat 1966;118(3):755–67.

7. Sarnat BG, Wexler MR. The snout after resection of nasal septum in adult rabbits. Arch Otolaryngol 1967;86:463–6.

8. Hartshorn DF. Facial growth effects of nasal septal cartilage resection in beagle pups. Iowa City (IA): University of Iowa Press; 1970.

9. Squier CA, Wada T, Ghoneim S, et al. A histological and ultrastructural study of wound healing after vomer resection in the beagle dog. Arch Oral Biol 1985;30(11–12):833–41.

10. Stenström SJ, Thilander BL. Effects of nasal septal cartilage resections on young guinea pigs. Plast Reconstr Surg 1970;45(2):160–70.

11. Fuchs P. Experimental production of growth disturbance by using a caudally based vomerine flap in rabbits. Amsterdam: Excerpta Medical Foundation; 1969. p. 484–8.

12. Bernstein L. Early submucous resection of nasal septal cartilage. A pilot study in canine pups. Arch Otolaryngol 1973;97:273–8.

13. Cupero TM, Middleto CE, Silva AB. Effects of functional septoplasty on the facial growth of ferrets. Arch Otolaryngol Head Neck Surg 2001;127:1367–9.

14. Verwoerd CDA, Verwoerd-Verhoef HL. Rhinosurgery in children: basic concepts. Facial Plast Surg 2007; 23:219–30.

15. Nolst Trenité GJ. Rhinoplasty in children. In: Papel ID, Frodel JL, Larrabee WF, editors. Facial plastic and reconstructive surgery. 3rd edition. New York: Thieme; 2009. p. 605–17.

16. Bae JS, Kim ES, Jang YJ. Treatment outcomes of pediatric rhinoplasty: the Asan Medical Center experience. Int J Mediator Otorhinolaryngol 2013; 77:1701–10.

17. Christophel JJ, Gross CW. Pediatric septoplasty. Otolaryngol Clin North Am 2009;42:287–94.

18. Van Loosen J, Verwoerd-Verhoef HL, Verwoerd CD. The nasal septal cartilage in the newborn. Rhinology 1988;26:161–5.

19. Poublon RM, Verwoerd CD, Verwoerd-Verhoef HL. Anatomy of the upper lateral cartilages in the human newborn. Rhinology 1990;28:41–5.

20. Van Loosen J, Van Zanten GA, Howard CV, et al. Growth characteristics of the human nasal septum. Rhinology 1996;34(2):78–82.

21. Zankl A, Eberle L, Molinari L, et al. Growth charts for nose length, nasal protrusion and philtrum length from birth to 97 years. Am J Med Genet 2002;111: 388–91.

22. Dispenza F, Saraniti C, Sciandra D, et al. Management of naso-septal deformity in childhood: long-term results. Auris Nasus Larynx 2009;36:665–70.

23. Linder-Aronson S. Adenoids: their effect on mode of breathing and nasal airflow and their relationship to characteristics of the facial skeleton and the dentition: a biometric, rhino-manometric and cephalometro-radiographic study on children with and without adenoids. Acta Otolaryngol Suppl 1970;265:1–132.

24. Principato JJ. Upper airway obstruction and craniofacial morphology. Otolaryngol Head Neck Surg 1991;104(6):881–90.

25. Josell SD. Habits affecting dental and maxillofacial growth and development. Dent Clin North Am 1995;39(4):851–60.

26. Valera FCP, Travitzki LVV, Mattar SEM, et al. Muscular, functional and orthodontic changes in preschool children with enlarged adenoids and tonsils. Int J Pediatr Otorhinolaryngol 2003;67(7): 761–70.

27. Pirsig W, Lehmann I. The influence of trauma on the growing septal cartilage. Rhinology 1975;13(1):39–46.

28. Tasca I, Compadretti GC. Nasal growth after pediatric septoplasty at long-term follow-up. Am J Rhioln Allergy 2011;25(1):e7–12.

29. Harari D, Redlich M, Miri S, et al. The effect of mouth breathing versus nasal breathing on dentofacial and craniofacial development in orthodontic patients. Laryngoscope 2010;120(10):2089–93.

30. Adil E, Goyal N, Fedok FG. Corrective nasal surgery in the younger patient. JAMA Facial Plast Surg 2014; 16(3):176–82.

31. Crysdale WS. Nasal surgery in children: a personal perspective. J Otolaryngol Head Neck Surg 2009; 38(2):183–90.

32. O'Connor-Reina C, Garcia-Iriarte MT, Angel DG, et al. Radiofrequency volumetric tissue reduction for treatment of turbinate hypertrophy in children. Int J Pediatr Otorhinolaryngol 2007;71:597–601.

33. Chen YL, Liu CM, Huang HM. Comparison of microdebrider-assisted inferior turbinoplasty and submucosal resection for children with hypertrophic inferior turbinates. Int J Pediatr Otorhinolaryngol 2007;71:921–7.

34. Sullivan S, Li K, Guilleminault C. Nasal obstruction in children with sleep disordered breathing. Ann Acad Med Singapore 2008;37:645–8.

35. Leong SC, Kubba H, White PS. A review of outcomes following inferior turbinate reduction surgery in children for chronic nasal obstruction. Int J Pediatr Otorhinolaryngol 2010;74:1–6.

36. Jiang ZY, Pereira KD, Friedman NR, et al. Inferior turbinate surgery in children: a survey of practice patterns. Laryngoscope 2012;122: 1620–3.

37. Lawrence R. Pediatric septoplasty: a review of the literature. Int J Pediatr Otorhinolaryngol 2012;76: 1078–81.

38. D'Ascanio L, Lancione C, Pompa G, et al. Craniofacial growth in children with nasal septum deviation: a cephalometric comparative study. Int J Pediatr Otorhinolaryngol 2010;74:1180–3.

39. El-Hakim H, Crysdale WS, Abdollel M, et al. A study of anthropometric measures before and after external septoplasty in children: a preliminary study. Arch Otolaryngol Head Neck Surg 2001; 127:1362–6.

40. Liu C, Legocki AT, Mader NS, et al. Nasal Fractures in children and adolescents: Mechanisms of injury and efficacy of closed reduction. Int J Pediatr Otorhinolaryngol 2015;79(12):2238–42.

41. Desrosiers AE, Thaller SR. Pediatric nasal fractures: evaluation and management. J Craniofac Surg 2011;22:1327–9.

42. Zimmermann CE, Troulis MJ, Kaban LB. Pediatric facial fractures: recent advances in prevention, diagnosis and management. Int J Oral Maxillofac Surg 2006;35(1):2–13.

43. Precious DS, Delaire J, Hoffman CD. The effects of nasomaxillary injury on future facial growth. Oral Surg Oral Med Oral Pathol 1988;66:525–30.

44. Moran WB. Nasal trauma in children. Otolaryngol Clin North Am 1977;10:95–101.

45. Higuera S, Lee EI, Stal S. Nasal trauma and the deviated nose. Plast Reconstr Surg 2007;120(7,suppl 2): 64S–75S.

46. Wright RJ, Murakami CS, Ambro BT. Pediatric nasal injuries and management. Facial Plast Surg 2011; 27:483–90.

47. Canty PA, Berkowitz RG. Haematoma and abscess of the nasal septum in children. Arch Otolaryngol Head Neck Surg 1996;122:1373–6.

48. Zielnik-Jurkiewicz B, Olszewska-Sosińska O, Rapiejko P. Treatment of the nasal septal hematoma and abscess in children. Otolaryngol Pol 2008;62: 71–5.

49. Alshaikh N, Lo S. Nasal septal abscess in children: from diagnosis to management and prevention. Int J Pediatr Otorhinolaryngol 2011;75:737–44.

50. Jalaludin MA. Nasal septal abscess: retrospective analysis of 14 cases from university hospital. Kulalumpur Singapore Med J 1993;34:435–7.

51. Matsuba HM, Thawley SE. Nasal septal abscess: unusual causes, complications, treatment and sequelae. Ann Plast Surg 1986;16:161–6.

52. Dennis SCR, den Herder C, Shandilya M, et al. Open rhinoplasty in children. Facial Plast Surg 2007;23: 259–66.

53. Menger DJ, Tabink IC, Trenité GJ. Nasal septal abscess in children: reconstruction with autologous cartilage grafts on polydioxanone plate. Arch Otolaryngol Head Neck Surg 2008;134:842–7.

54. Hellmich S. Reconstruction of the destroyed septal infrastructure. Otolaryngol Head Neck Surg 1989; 100:92–4.

55. Close DM, Guinness MD. Abscess of the nasal septum after trauma. Med J Aust 1985;142:472–4.

56. Lee TS, Schwartz GM, Tatum SA. Rhinoplasty for cleft and hemangioma-related nasal deformities. Curr Opin Otolaryngol Head Neck Surg 2010; 18(6):526–35.

57. Liou EJW, Subramanian M, Chen PKT, et al. The progressive changes of nasal symmety and growth after nasoalveolar molding: a three-year follow up study. Plast Reconstr Surg 2004;114(4):858–64.

58. Jones LR, Tatum SA. Pearls for aesthetic reconstruction of cleft lip and nose defects. Facial Plast Surg 2008;24(1):146–51.

59. Sykes JM, Senders CW. Surgery of the cleft lip and nasal deformity. Oper Tech Otolaryngol Head Neck Surg 1990;1:219–24.

60. Sykes JM. The importance of primary rhinoplasty at the time of initial unilateral cleft lip repair. Arch Facial Plast Surg 2010;12(1):53–5.

61. Pawar SS, Wang TD. Secondary cleft rhinoplasty. JAMA Facial Plast Surg 2014;16(1):58–63.

62. Bhattacharjee A, Uddin S, Purkaystha P. Deviated nasal septum in the newborn - A 1 year study. Ind J Otolaryngol Head Neck Surg 2005;57(4): 304–8.

63. Chintapatla S, Kudva YC, Nayar RC, et al. Septal deviation in neonates. Indian Pediatr 1989;26: 678–82.

64. Gray LP. The deviated nasal septum. Aetiology J Laryngol Otol 1965;79:567–75.

65. Jazbi B. Diagnosis and treatment of nasal birth deformities. Clin Paediatr 1974;13:1974.

66. Emami AJ, Brodsky L, Pizzuto M. Neonatal septoplasty: case report and review of the literature. Int J Pediatr Otorhinolaryngol 1996;35(3):271–5.

67. Fior R, Veljak C. Septum dislocation in the newborn: a long term followup study of immediate reposition. Rhinology 1990;28:159–62.

68. Jazbi B. Subluxation of the nasal septum in the newborn: etiology, diagnosis and treatment. Otolaryngol Clin North Am 1977;10:125–38.

69. Healy G. An approach to the nasal septum in children. Laryngoscope 1986;96:1239–42.

70. Ortiz-Monasterio F, Olmedo A. Corrective rhinoplasty before puberty: a long-term follow-up. Plast Reconstr Surg 1981;68:381–91.

71. Bejar I, Farkas LG, Messner AH, et al. Nasal growth after external septoplasty in children. Arch Otolaryngol Head Neck Surg 1996;122: 816–21.

72. McComb HK, Coghlan BA. Primary repair of the unilateral cleft lip nose: completion of a longitudinal study. Cleft Palate Craniofac J 1996;33: 23–30.

Cleft Septorhinoplasty
Form and Function

Tsung-yen Hsieh, MD[a], Raj Dedhia, MD[a], Drew Del Toro, BSc[a],
Travis T. Tollefson, MD, MPH[b],*

KEYWORDS

- Cleft lip nasal deformity • Cleft lip rhinoplasty • Presurgical infant orthopedics
- Nasoalveolar molding • Primary cleft lip rhinoplasty • Secondary revision rhinoplasty

KEY POINTS

- Considered by many rhinoplasty surgeons to be the most difficult to master, cleft lip septorhinoplasty is a challenge requiring understanding of the primary deformity and lip/nose repairs in infancy.
- Surgical planning to address the typical characteristics incorporate the typical grafting and suture techniques used in noncleft rhinoplasty, but adept use of cleft-specific techniques is required (alar hooding, alar base asymmetry, columellar shortening, deficiency in the piriform/premaxilla, and nostril shape).
- Skeletal disproportion from the cleft deformity plays a major role in the nasal deformity. Ideally the bony deficit is treated with appropriately timed alveolar cleft and premaxillary bone grafting.
- Septal or rib cartilage grafts should be used to create a stable caudal septal projection. The lower lateral cartilages are then set into position to the rotation and projection of choice using a tongue-in-groove technique.
- Thick-skinned nasal tips require conservative soft tissue debulking or soft tissue envelope thinning to improve tip contour and definition.

INTRODUCTION

Cleft lip and/or palate formation is the most common congenital craniofacial abnormality, constituting 1 in 500 to 1000 live births.[1] Some variability in ethnicity has been noted, with higher incidence in Native Americans and Asian populations,[2] and lower incidence in African Americans and Africans.[3] Orofacial clefting seems to be multifactorial, associated with genetics and environmental factors.[4]

The nasal deformity associated with typical cleft lip can result in significant aesthetic and functional issues that can be difficult to address. The nasal deformity has classic descriptions for the unilateral (**Box 1**) and bilateral (**Box 2**) cleft lip, but the nasal findings occur with significant variability along a spectrum of severity. The nose's central position has an important role in facial aesthetics and the perception of normal facial features.[5] In cleft nasal deformity the distortion of the nose can range from minimal to severe,[6] emphasizing the importance of a patient-centered approach to repair. In order to maximize function and appearance through cleft septorhinoplasty, it is crucial to understand the embryologic origin of clefting and the anatomic structure in nasal cleft deformity.

This article reviews cleft lip nasal deformity, presurgical care, primary cleft rhinoplasty, and

Disclosures: None of the authors has any financial or other disclosures with regard to this article.
[a] Department of Otolaryngology-Head and Neck Surgery, UC Davis Medical Center, 2521 Stockton Boulevard, Suite 7200, Sacramento, CA 95817, USA; [b] Facial Plastic and Reconstructive Surgery, Department of Otolaryngology-Head and Neck Surgery, UC Davis Medical Center, 2521 Stockton Boulevard, Suite 7200, Sacramento, CA 95817, USA
* Corresponding author.
E-mail address: tttollefson@ucdavis.edu

Facial Plast Surg Clin N Am 25 (2017) 223–238
http://dx.doi.org/10.1016/j.fsc.2016.12.011

Box 1
Characteristics of unilateral cleft lip nasal deformity

- Grossly asymmetric
- Nose has longer appearance on cleft side
- Retrodisplaced cleft-side dome
- Base of columella deviated toward noncleft side
- Nostril is wider and retrodisplaced on cleft side
- Nostril margin on cleft side buckles inward because of bowing by internal vestibular web
- Deficient maxilla on cleft side (often absent nasal floor affecting piriform aperture)
- Posterolaterally displaced alar base and piriform margin on cleft side
- Anterolaterally displaced anterior nasal spine
- Deviated premaxilla, columella, and caudal septum toward noncleft side
- Posterolaterally displaced cleft-side dome of lower lateral cartilage (LLC)
- Increased angle between medial and lateral crura on cleft side
- Short medial crus on cleft side
- Long lateral crus on cleft side
- Upper lateral cartilage and LLC on cleft side are side by side rather than normal overlap

Adapted from Cuzalina A, Jung C. Rhinoplasty for the cleft lip and palate patient. Oral Maxillofac Surg Clin North Am 2016;28(2):189–202.

Box 2
Characteristics of bilateral cleft lip nasal deformity

- Grossly symmetric
- Wide nose with broad and depressed tip
- Short columella
- Wide nostrils with inward collapsing margins
- Flared alae with bilateral vestibular webbing
- Posterolaterally displaced alar domes
- Increased angles of divergence between the medial and lateral crura
- Shortened medial crura
- Longer lateral crura
- Protrusive premaxilla
- Hypoplastic maxilla bilaterally
- Anterior nasal spine and caudal septum are inferiorly displaced relative to the alar bases
- Deficient or absent bony nasal floor

Adapted from Cuzalina A, Jung C. Rhinoplasty for the cleft lip and palate patient. Oral Maxillofac Surg Clin North Am 2016;28(2):189–202.

the development, as the CNC continues to migrate into the maxillary prominences, the medial and lateral nasal prominence join the premaxillary segment to form the nares, nasal tip, and philtral column (**Fig. 1**).

This coordinated process involves a multitude of transcription factors, and regulation of growth signals. Disruption of the transcriptional or growth factor signals in development results in malformations of the upper lip, central alveolus, and/or the primary palate,[8] including clefting of the lip and palate. Extent of cleft nasal deformity is associated with extent of interruption of the normal development, with a spectrum of varying severity of lip and associated nasal deformities. However, even when subtle, nasal deformities are always associated with cleft lips.[10]

ANATOMIC DEFORMITY

Nasal deformity associated with unilateral and bilateral cleft have been well documented. Understanding the consistent skeletal and muscular dysmorphism and asymmetry is essential in providing the most cosmetic and functional repair.

Unilateral Cleft Lip Nasal Deformity and Dysfunction

In unilateral cleft lip nasal deformity, there are several well-described characteristics (see

definitive cleft septorhinoplasty, with a focus on restoring symmetry and contour to the shape, and maintaining or improving function.

EMBRYOLOGY

During embryologic development, the upper lip formation begins at approximately 4 weeks of gestation with completion at 3 to 4 months of gestation.[7] Most facial skeleton and connective tissue is developed from a pluripotent population of cells and cranial neural crest (CNC) cells that show remarkable migratory abilities as well as ability for development into diverse cell types.[8] Migration of the CNC cells into the frontonasal prominence facilitates the formation of the forehead, nasal dorsum, median and lateral nasal prominences, premaxilla, and the philtrum.[9] This highly regulated process starts with paired bilateral maxillary prominences, derived from the first branchial arches, merging toward the midline to form the lateral aspect of the upper lip. Later in

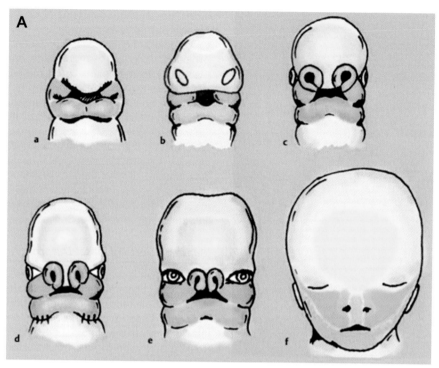

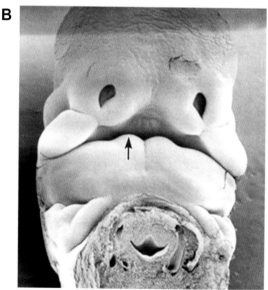

Fig. 1. (*A*) Human craniofacial development illustrated with embryos shown at 4, 5, 5.5, and 6 weeks and term infant from top to bottom. Six facial prominences are color coded: blue, mandibular; orange, maxillary; pink, lateral nasal; green, medial nasal; and yellow, frontal. (*B*) Scanning electron microscopic view of an embryo early in development of the merging medial nasal prominences (*arrow*). In this *Macaca fascicularis* embryo, all the lateral nasal, medial nasal, maxillary, frontonasal, and mandibular prominences are seen. (*Courtesy of* [A] Amir Rafii, MD, Sacramento, CA; and *From* Senders CW, Peterson EC, Hendrickx AG, et al. Development of the upper lip. Arch Facial Plast Surg 2003;5(1):16–25; with permission.)

Box 1). There is asymmetry of the nasal tip and alar base caused by a deficiency of the maxilla on the cleft side[11] (**Fig. 2**). As a result, the cleft-side alar base does not merge in the midline, which contributes to the classically described unilateral cleft lip nasal deformity. These soft tissue asymmetries as well as the maxillary skeletal deficiency leave the cleft-side alar base more posterior, inferior, and lateral compared with the noncleft side.[12,13]

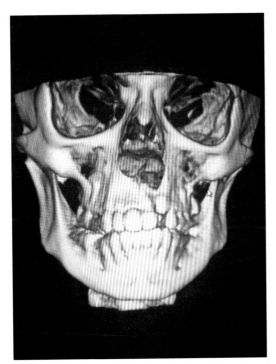

Fig. 2. Computed tomography three-dimensional reconstruction image showing deficient nasal floor on the left of a patient with unilateral cleft lip deformity.

The nasal tip asymmetry is caused by a dysmorphic shape of the cleft-side lower lateral cartilage (LLC). The cleft-side LLC has a short medial crus and a long lateral crus compared with the noncleft side. The asymmetry of the LLC and subsequent muscle pull generates a wide and horizontally oriented nostril.[14,15] There is also discontinuity of the orbicularis oris on the cleft side and improper insertion into the columella on the noncleft side, which pulls the columella and caudal septum toward the noncleft side, with resultant posterior, lateral, and inferior displacement of the alar base on the cleft side.[10] The nasal septum is then deviated toward the noncleft side caudally and bows dorsally toward the cleft side.[11] In addition, the attachment of the upper lateral cartilage is affected by the irregularity of the LLC, which weakens the scroll region and compromises the internal nasal valve[9] (**Fig. 3**).

Bilateral Cleft Lip Nasal Deformity

Bilateral cleft lip nasal deformity shares many features with unilateral cleft lip nasal deformity but is grossly symmetric rather than asymmetric (see **Box 2**).[11] There is often bony deficiency medially and inferiorly at the piriform of the maxilla. The premaxilla and overlying prolabium extend from the nasal septum in the complete bilateral cleft lip (a key point is that the amount of prolabial soft tissue is a key factor to the primary repair and the resulting nasal deformity). The alar bases are more posterior, inferior, and lateral in position. An underprojection of the nasal tip has been suggested to occur because of longer lateral crura and shorter medial crura of the LLC.[16] The authors believe that the

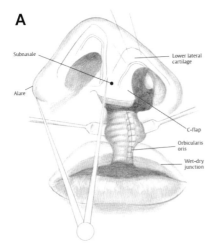

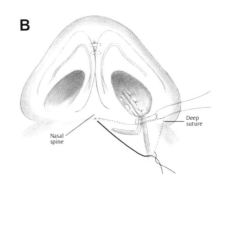

Fig. 3. Unilateral cleft nasal deformity. (*A*) During repair, the orbicularis oris muscle edges are brought together to establish dynamic lip movement and volume. A caliper is shown measuring the alar base on the normal side, which is compared with the alar base on the cleft side. The cleft-side alar base is set to the alar base width either symmetric or slightly narrower than the noncleft side (nasal floor creation should include excess mucosa and epithelium to prevent nasal stenosis). (*B*) The cleft-side LLC is to be repositioned into more normal anatomic position with sutures. The alar base "cinching" or "key" suture is placed between the periosteum near the nasal spine and soft tissues posterior to the alar base. (*From* Tollefson TT, Sykes JM. Unilateral cleft lip. In: Goudy S, Tollefson TT, editors. Complete cleft care. New York: Thieme; 2015. p. 55; with permission.)

cartilage deformation of the LLCs includes nearly normal cartilage volume and size, but differences in how the cartilages are folded caused by the abnormal muscle attachments and distribution of forces caused by the bilateral cleft lip.

A broad and flat nasal tip with hooding of the alae are seen. Malpositioning of the prolabium and shortened medial crura results in a short columella with a wide base, which makes the nasal tip lack even more definition.[7,11] The insertion of the orbicularis oris bilaterally into the alar base adds further to nasal alar base widening, which worsens with facial animation. The nasal septum is generally midline; however, if there is any asymmetry, the septum deviates toward the less affected side, where the muscle attachments are pulling the caudal septum.[17,18] External and internal nasal valves can be affected because of poor upper lateral cartilage and LLC strength, which has potential to cause nasal breathing difficulties with valve collapse.[19] Curvature of the lateral-most LLCs can create folds of redundant internal nasal valve nasal lining, also called plica vestibularis[7] (**Fig. 4**).

PRESURGICAL MANAGEMENT

Before surgical repair, patients with wide, complete cleft lip-palate may benefit from presurgical infant orthopedics (PSIO), which include appliances that can reposition the maxillary and nasal structures in more anatomic positions and allow for less wound tension after surgical repair, with the goal of potentially improving outcomes after primary repair (**Fig. 5**).

Nasoalveolar Molding

Manipulation of the premaxilla before surgical repair for cleft lip and palate has been reported since the sixteenth century.[20] Initially this included lip taping, elastics, orthodontics, and acrylic appliances. These devices were collectively referred to as PSIO. Over the years, maxillary arch devices were developed that connected the protruding premaxilla with lateral arch segments.[21,22] Another option is the Latham device, which is used to shift the premaxilla and lateral alveolar segments by using a pin-retained appliance.[23,24] The modern nasoalveolar molding (NAM) appliance was created by Grayson and colleagues.[25] It combines an orthodontic device on the premaxilla and lateral alveolar segments with nasal stents. The device is fitted to the maxilla with molding and the stents are then fixed in place with taping.

After the introduction of NAM therapy, Grayson and Cutting[26] noted improved appearance of the nose with a reduction in secondary nasal surgeries and decreased need for alveolar bone grafting.[20,26] An oral appliance, such as the Hotz appliance or Zurich plates, functions as a static palatal plate once adapted to the cleft alveolus. The presence of increased serum maternal estrogen level allows nasal cartilages to be more readily corrected. The cartilage is made more flexible by the release of proteoglycans and hyaluronic acid caused by increased estrogen levels. The hormones that contribute to the increased elasticity of cartilage in a mother's pelvis also is thought to affect a neonate's ear and nasal cartilages.[27,28] In addition, studies by Matsuo and colleagues[29]

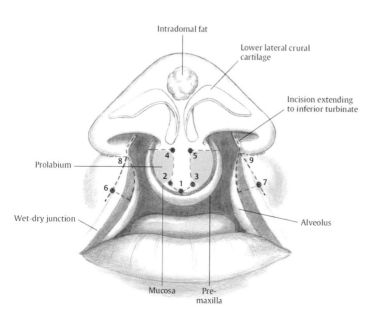

Fig. 4. Bilateral cleft nasal deformity. The design of the prolabial skin, which creates a narrow philtrum. This will grow under the lateral tension created by the lip repair to create an anthropometrically normal philtral subunit after facial growth. The numbered dots represent lip markings for surgical planning. (*From* Tollefson TT, Sykes JM. Unilateral cleft lip. In: Goudy S, Tollefson TT, editors. Complete cleft care. New York: Thieme; 2015. p. 74; with permission.)

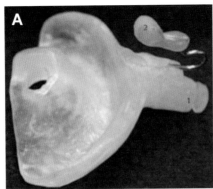
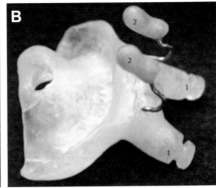

Fig. 5. (*A*) Unilateral nasoalveolar molding (NAM) appliance, with retention button (1) and nasal stent (2). (*B*) Bilateral NAM appliance, with 2 retention buttons (1) and 2 nasal stents (2). Note that the 2 nasal stents will be connected following addition of the horizontal columella band. (*From* Garfinkle JS, Kapadia H. Presurgical treatment. In: Goudy S, Tollefson TT, editors. Complete cleft care. New York: Thieme; 2015. p. 13; with permission.)

also showed the ability of infant auricular cartilage to be molded.[29]

The goal of NAM therapy is to bring the maxillary segments together and, in cases of bilateral cleft, to retract the premaxilla posteriorly to approximate the level of the maxillary segments. In addition, the nasal prongs serve the purpose of bringing the lip segments together, elongate the columella in the bilateral cleft, expand the nasal mucosal lining, and mold the lower lateral alar cartilages to more symmetric positions.[25]

In infants with bilateral cleft, the lateral alveolar clefts are moved medially and the protruding premaxilla is moved medially and posteriorly. Next, nasal stents are applied to the retention arms with a soft denture material added to serve as a bridge between the 2 sides (**Fig. 6**). The bridge functions as a nonsurgical method to lengthen the columella, which helps define the nasolabial

junction. Applying gentle pressure to this area can also facilitate lengthening of the prolabium. As a result, the need for secondary columellar lengthening is reduced.[26]

Evidence-Based Approach to Presurgical Infant Orthopedics

Use of PSIO is highly debated. The long-term outcomes of NAM therapy before primary surgical repair are controversial. Contributing factors to the controversy over NAM include a lack of clear objective outcome assessments, discrepancies in techniques used between cleft centers, and an ever-changing measure of success.[30] Systematic reviews have not been able to identify negative impacts of PSIO, excluding NAM. There is also insufficient evidence of potential primary benefits such as ultimate facial growth, maxillary form, dental

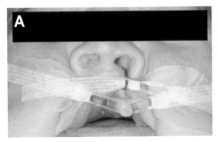
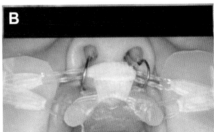

Fig. 6. Face tapes and the NAM appliance. (*A*) Taping for unilateral cleft lip and palate (UCLP). Base tapes are applied to the cheeks. The appliance is then inserted and the retention tapes are secured to the retention button. Greater tension can be placed on the side with the cleft to favor alveolar cleft closure. A cross-cheek tape can be added to provide additional force as described in the text. (*B*) Taping for bilateral cleft lip and palate. The taping is similar to the UCLP except each retention tape inserts on the retention button on its respective side. Differential force can be placed on each tape to address any premaxillary deviation. A prolabial tape can be added to facilitate nonsurgical columella elongation. Lip taping can be added to provide additional force for premaxillary retraction as described in the text. (*From* Garfinkle JS, Kapadia H. Presurgical treatment. In: Goudy S, Tollefson TT, editors. Complete cleft care. New York: Thieme; 2015. p. 13; with permission.)

occlusion, or speech, and potential secondary benefits such as parental satisfaction or improvement in feeding (level II evidence).[31,32]

Opponents of NAM propose that midface growth and dental arch shape may be inhibited by moving the maxillary segments. Furthermore, they suggest that nasal improvements have a significant rate of relapse. A 10% to 20% relapse rate in nostril width and height has been reported after NAM and unilateral cleft lip repair in the first year.[33] However, this relapse could be countered by overcorrecting the cleft-side nostril.[28,34]

In 2012, Abbott and Meara[35] published a review supporting the effectiveness of NAM on the nasal form in unilateral cleft lip (level III evidence). After reviewing the evidence (levels II–V), the investigators concluded that although negative effects were unlikely, benefits in bilateral cleft deformity were also unclear. This lack of clarity is in part caused by a lack of well-designed and controlled outcomes assessments. The confounding variables in the studies reviewed, such as inconsistency in techniques of NAM and lip repair, degree of cleft severity, and the need for a long duration of follow-up, are difficult to control. In the future, studies should aim to incorporate multiple sites, rigid inclusion criteria, rigorous controls, and a multidisciplinary approach.

At present, in our practice, NAM is used in both unilateral and bilateral cleft repair with strong consideration of the socioeconomic impact on parents (ie, residing a long distance from a cleft center), parental compliance, and cleft severity.[36,37]

PRIMARY CLEFT RHINOPLASTY

Primary cleft rhinoplasty at the time of the cleft lip repair has become a more common practice since the 1970s, and has been shown to reduce the severity of deformity and the number of revision surgeries required in adulthood.[38] It is important to ensure symmetry during the initial surgery because any asymmetry becomes more apparent with growth. However, care must be taken to avoid excessive dissection to prevent future scarring or stenosis that may complicate the secondary rhinoplasty.

In unilateral cleft nasal deformity, the goal of the primary rhinoplasty is to restore nasal tip symmetry, and correct excessive alar hooding on the cleft side. In bilateral cleft nasal deformity, the primary rhinoplasty serves to reduce alar flare, correct malpositioning of the LLC, reconstruct the nasal sills, restore projection of the nasal tip, and augment the columellar length.[39–41]

In primary rhinoplasty for unilateral cleft lip nasal deformity, blunt dissection of the LLCs from the soft tissue envelope is done through the columellar lip incision. The cleft-side LLC can then be positioned in a more cephalad and medial position either using a Skoog technique or triangular fixation sutures. The Skoog technique involves an intracartilaginous or marginal rhinoplasty incision for access and suturing the cleft-side LLC to the upper lateral cartilage and septum (**Fig. 7**).

The senior author prefers to use the triangular fixation sutures using resorbable 5-0 Monocryl sutures. These sutures are placed transnasally out to the alar crease and back into the nose while the nasal tip and cleft-side LLC is pressed cephalad with a Brown forceps placed inside the nostril, passing a needle from the vestibular surface through the alar crease to the noncleft-side nasal tip and back in the needle hole while holding the cleft-side LLC in position. The suture is then tied within the nose (**Fig. 8**). In cases of severe nostril hooding, an elliptical excision of the soft tissue hooding, Tajima reverse-U rim incision, can be made with interdomal sutures (5-0 polydioxanone sutures) placed through this incision. The cleft-side alar base is repositioned symmetrically with the noncleft alar base with an alar base cinching suture. The nasal sill edges are then reapproximated using absorbable sutures, placed as far posterior as possible.

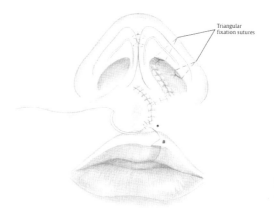

Fig. 7. Transcutaneous plication sutures are passed first from inside the nose, through the nasal lining, LLC, and out the skin. The needle is then passed back through the dermal hold that it just came through and passed at a different trajectory inside the nose. The absorbable (Monocryl 5-0) suture is tied inside the nostril. Final skin closure with triangle flaps just above the white roll (*asterisk*) and at the Noordhoff red line (*hash symbol*) (eg, the wet-dry junction of the red lip). Typically, subcutaneous sutures are used to minimize suture marks. (*From* Tollefson TT, Sykes JM. Unilateral cleft lip. In: Goudy S, Tollefson TT, editors. Complete cleft care. New York: Thieme; 2015. p. 56; with permission.)

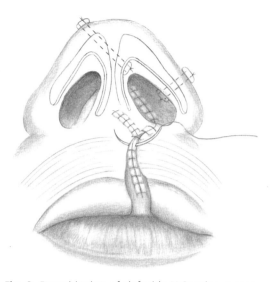

Fig. 8. Repositioning of cleft-side LLCs using suspension sutures that are placed through and through the nasal skin and nasal-vestibular lining. (*From* Tollefson TT, Sykes JM. Unilateral cleft lip. In: Goudy S, Tollefson TT, editors. Complete cleft care. New York: Thieme; 2015; with permission.)

For bilateral cleft lip, the nasal tip fat pad is first exposed via bilateral partial marginal incisions. Excess fibrofatty tissue between the LLCs is excised. The LLCs are then sewn together in the midline in a lateral crural steal maneuver, to improve projection of the nasal tip. The cephalic borders of the LLCs are secured cephalad onto the upper lateral cartilages. Tajima reverse U can again be completed if there is excessive hooding. The nasal floor is closed with 5-0 chromic and the alar base cinching suture is placed with 4-0 Vicryl or polydioxanone to narrow the interalar distances to less than 25 mm. The alar bases on each side are sutured to the underlying orbicularis oris muscle to allow better positioning of the lateral nasal sill. The columellar elongation is required in rare cases, and recruiting tissue from the lip through a V-Y columellar elongation or forked flap procedure can be accomplished.

At the conclusion of the primary cleft rhinoplasty, the caudal septum is secured with nasal conformers, which serve to stent open the collapsed nostrils and support the primary rhinoplasty maneuvers for up to 6 weeks (**Fig. 9**). Care should be taken not to blanch the skin on the nasal tip from the conformers.[42]

SECONDARY CLEFT SEPTORHINOPLASTY
Intermediate Rhinoplasty

Classically, some surgeons preferred to address the nasal deformity at the time of the primary cleft lip repair, waiting for an intermediate rhinoplasty (after the primary lip repair but before a definitive

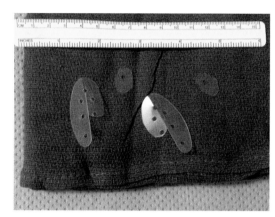

Fig. 9. Nasal stent. Modified Reuter-Bobbin septal splints to be placed in internal nasal valve and secured with transalar suture with external suture. These splints stent the valve open, compress the alar grafts, and are removed after 7 to 10 days.

rhinoplasty at full skeletal development). Examples include the use of a secondary columellar lengthening with a V-Y advancement, often completed with nasal tip intradomal sutures and transdomal fat transposition or removal. The senior author prefers to address the rhinoplasty at the neonatal stage and reserves intermediate rhinoplasty techniques for nasal obstruction from cleft-side plica vestibularis or thickening of the alar (occluding the airway.) A Z-plasty of this fold of intranasal mucosa and skin with or without a small septal lateral crural strut graft is effective for this problem (**Fig. 10**).

Definitive Rhinoplasty

Secondary (definitive) cleft rhinoplasty is performed once facial skeletal maturity is reached. Cartilage grafting material from the rib or septum is usually needed for structural reconstruction of the cleft nose to achieve adequate support. The goals of secondary cleft septorhinoplasty are to create symmetry and definition of the nasal base and tip; relieve nasal obstruction; and repair nasal scarring, nasal stenosis, and webbing. The degree of secondary nasal deformity can be diverse. Several factors affect this variability and include the degree of the original lip and nose defect, surgeries completed before secondary cleft rhinoplasty, and differences in nasal growth.[43] The definitive cleft septorhinoplasty therefore is tailored to individual patients. This procedure is usually performed after completion of nasal and midfacial growth, around age 14 to 16 years in girls and 16 to 18 years in boys.

Surgical Approach

An external or endonasal approach to secondary cleft rhinoplasty often depends on surgeon

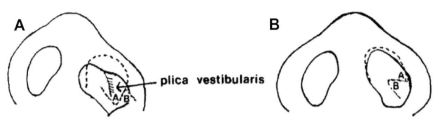

plica vestibularis

Fig. 10. The recurvature of the cleft-side LLC and plica vestibularis can be treated with a Z-plasty modification of the Tajima reverse-U incision. Lateral wall Z-plasty introduces additional internal lining to the cleft-side vestibule. It also provides a larger incision in the lateral vestibule for access to place the suspension sutures. A and B in the figures represent the two triangular flaps created during the Z-plasty that are transposed. (*A*) Suture lines. (*B*) final closure after transposition of flaps. (*From* Nakajima T, Yoshimura Y, Kami T. Refinement of the "reverse-U" incision for the repair of cleft lip nose deformity. Br J Plast Surg 1986;39(3):345–51; with permission.)

preference and the requirements of the reconstruction. The major factors that are contributing to the nasal deformity, including the need for septal reconstruction, and management of the nasal tip, alar rim, alar base, columella, and nasal sill, should be identified before surgery in order to determine the appropriate approach to achieve successful reconstruction. In addition, the previous cleft lip repair should be considered when determining the approach if further revision of the lip repair is required.

Alveolar Bone Grafting

Alveolar bone grafting and premaxilla advancement surgeries (Le Fort I osteotomy) have an important role in providing the skeleton for maxillary projection. This is important to be completed before definitive rhinoplasty to establish the bony foundation of the maxilla for repair.[44,45] Orthognathic surgery should be performed before definitive rhinoplasty, as shown in **Fig. 11**.

Reconstruction of the Nasal Septum and Dorsum

In order to perform a complete septal reconstruction, adequate exposure and total breakdown of the ligamentous attachments contributing to septal deviation must be achieved. Either an open or an endonasal approach can be used to manage the septum. In the open approach, the anterior septum is exposed after separating the ligaments connecting the medial crura. In the endonasal approach, the exposure needed for septal reconstruction is achieved by joining a complete transfixion incision to bilateral cartilaginous incisions.

In unilateral cleft, the caudal septum of the cleft nasal deformity is typically deviated toward the noncleft side because of unopposed muscle tension from the orbicularis oris as well as deficiency in the maxilla.[46] In our practice, the caudal septum is separated from the nasal spine, repositioned to the midline, and secured to the periosteum of the spine in the proper position in a swinging-door maneuver. If needed, an anterior inferior wedge can be resected to facilitate movement of the septum. In bilateral cleft, the septum tends to be midline with occasional mild deviation toward the more asymmetric lip, which may require further septal support.[46] In either case, deviations in the cartilage and bone can be removed leaving adequate dorsal and caudal struts for septal support (**Fig. 12**).

Caudal septal extension graft (fashioned from septal cartilage, costal cartilage, or ethmoid plate bone) is frequently used as septal structural support and for subsequent treatment of the nasal tip in both unilateral and bilateral cleft deformities. The caudal septal extension graft can be secured to the existing nasal septum through an end-to-end or side-to-end technique (**Fig. 13**).

If additional support for the caudal and dorsum septum is required, use of spreader grafts placed between the septum and the upper lateral cartilages can provide additional structure, correct dorsal external deviations, and increase the internal valve cross-sectional area for airway improvement.[47]

Less commonly, if the septal deviation is so severe that cartilage resection or repositioning is not able to achieve the desired outcome, extracorporeal septoplasty may be necessary. This procedure involves explantation of the nasal septum, reshaping the septal cartilage, reimplanting the septum, and securing the septum dorsally and caudally.[48]

With regard to the nasal dorsum, similar techniques for cosmetic or functional septorhinoplasty can be used. Lateral osteotomies can be done to reposition the bony pyramid. In addition, disarticulating the upper lateral cartilages from dorsal septum with placement of asymmetrically sized spreader grafts can straighten the curvature of the dorsal nasal septum and improve the nasal airway of the internal nasal valve.[49,50]

232

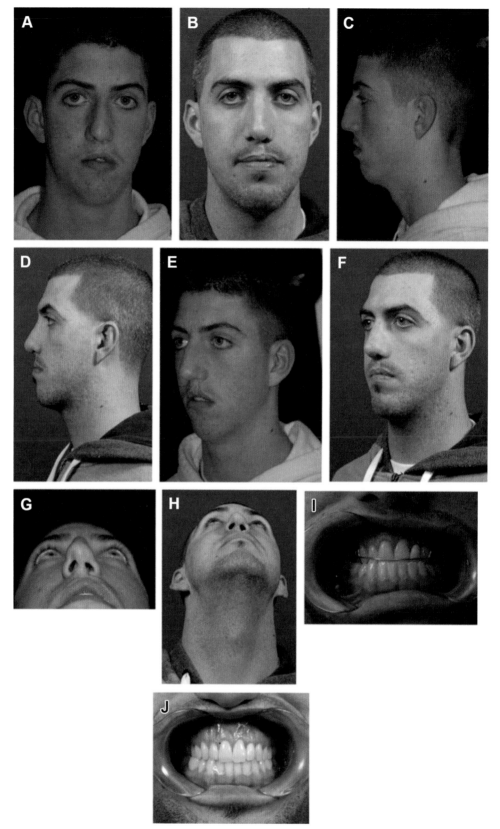

Fig. 11. Preoperative and postoperative views of patient with unilateral complete cleft lip and palate who underwent cleft septorhinoplasty that included asymmetric spreader grafts, caudal septal extension graft, alar rim grafts, lateral crural strut grafts, and alar base repositioning. (*A*) Preoperative and (*B*) 2-year postoperative

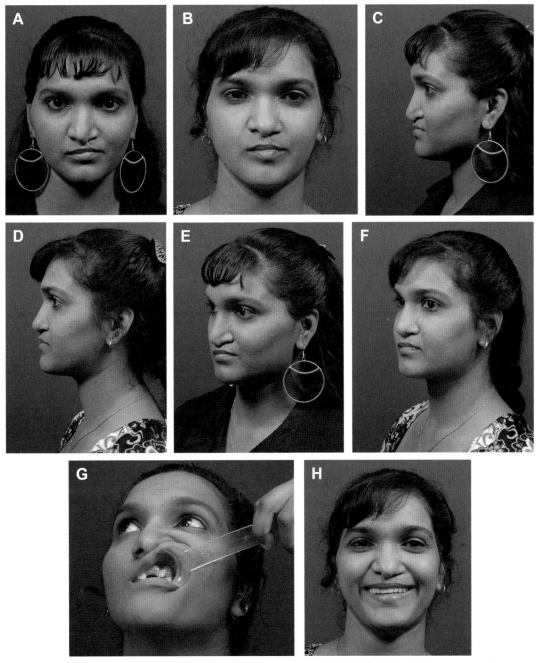

Fig. 12. A 25-year-old patient with unilateral complete cleft lip and palate after repair; however, she did not undergo primary cleft rhinoplasty, orthodontics, or alveolar cleft repair as a child. The left ala shows flattening, alar hooding, and grossly distorted intermediate crura of the LLC. Lack of tip definition is noted on the cleft side with caudal septal deviation to the noncleft (*right*) side. (*A*) Preoperative and (*B*) postoperative frontal views. (*C*) Preoperative and (*D*) postoperative lateral views. (*E*) Preoperative and (*F*) postoperative oblique views. (*G*) Preoperative intraoral view before alveolar bone grafting and extraction of severely decayed teeth and (*H*) frontal view showing smile with dental implants in place afterward.

frontal views. (*C*) Preoperative and (*D*) postoperative lateral views. (*E*) Preoperative and (*F*) postoperative oblique views. (*G*) Preoperative and (*H*) postoperative basal views. Dental occlusion shown (*I*) before and (*J*) after orthognathic surgery. (Rhinoplasty should be delayed until after orthognathic surgery at full skeletal growth.)

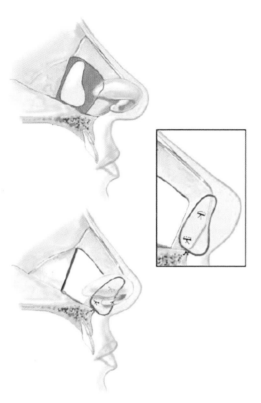

Fig. 13. Caudal septal extension graft. Cartilage graft placed side to end to the caudal septum. (*From* Toriumi DM. New concepts in tip contouring. Arch Facial Plast Surg 2006;8:166; with permission.)

Treatment of the Nasal Tip

In patients with congenital cleft lip, the nasal tip has poor support. As discussed previously, in unilateral cleft nasal deformity, the tip is asymmetric because of a shortened medial crus on the cleft side. In contrast, in bilateral cleft nasal deformity, there is poor support of the nasal tip and a short columella. Nasal tip treatment involves establishing symmetry, enhancing definition, and improving projection.

The tongue-in-groove (TIG) technique is frequently used to improve nasal tip support and projection. TIG involves resuspending the medial crura on the caudal nasal septum once the septum deformity has been straightened and supported. Placement of the sutures for resuspension with this technique can reshape, project, or deproject the nasal tip.[51] In unilateral cleft nasal deformities, the cleft-side nasal tip is usually underprojected with hooding of the ala, requiring projection and rotation for compensation. Applying the TIG technique, the cleft-side alar cartilage usually needs to be advanced more than the noncleft side to address the cleft LLC flattening and enhance nasal

tip symmetry. In bilateral cleft nasal deformity, a similar technique can be used to help project the nasal tip (**Fig. 14**).

Columellar strut grafts can often be used in management of the nasal tip. Cartilage graft harvested from septal cartilage, auricular cartilage, or costal chondral cartilage is placed between the medial crura of the LLCs to provide additional support and projection. The medial crural ligaments can be advanced and secured onto the strut graft to address symmetry, projection, and support. Furthermore, addition of a shield tip graft can further enhance the definition and projection of the nasal tip and to conceal irregularities, in situations in which the infratip lobule is insufficient.[50]

Lateral crural steal can also be accomplished by vertical domal division of the LLC. On the cleft side, the division is usually done lateral to the existing dome to provide additional length to the medial crura. Advancing and securing the medial

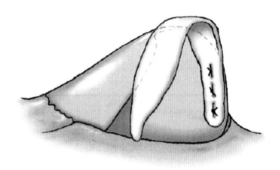

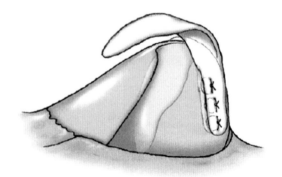

Fig. 14. TIG technique. The nasal tip is stabilized with a LLC (grafting lateral crural strut grafts, and either columellar strut or caudal septal extension grafts). The dome symmetry, projection, and rotation are then set using sutures placed between the medial crura (the groove in between the medial crus) and the septum or neoseptal grafting (the tongue). (*From* Kridel RWH, Scott BA, Foda HT. The tongue-in-groove technique in septorhinoplasty. Arch Facial Plast Surg 1999;1:249; with permission.)

crura using suspension sutures to septum or colu-mellar graft using techniques described earlier can improve the symmetry and projection of the nasal tip.[52] Again, addition of a tip graft can improve projection and definition, and camouflage tip irregularities.

Alar Rim

In unilateral cleft nasal deformity, the cleft-side lateral crus of the LLC is typically flattened because of alar malposition with inferior and pos-terior displacement of the cartilage relative to the noncleft-side LLC (**Fig. 15**). This concavity can result in external nasal valve collapse and func-tional deformity. In bilateral cleft nasal deformity, there can be symmetric flattening of alar rims that are poorly supported.

There are various techniques to correct the alar rim, including cartilage grafting and/or suture repositioning. Support for the cleft-side lateral crus can be achieved with alar rim grafts, alar strut grafts, alar turn-in flaps, or flip-flop of the LLC whereby an excision and turnover of the entire lateral crus of the LLC with resuturing of the segment is done.[53]

Cartilage grafts can be used to support the LLC. In the alar rim graft technique, a cartilage graft is placed inferior to the existing cartilage to provide additional strength to the alar rim. The alar strut graft involves placing a graft on the deep surface of the LLC with the graft sutured to the underside of the cartilage. The lateral extent of this graft is usually tucked into a precise pocket at the pyri-form aperture. In both of these grafts, the alar rim is supported in a manner that elevates the level of alar rim and repositions the rim laterally.

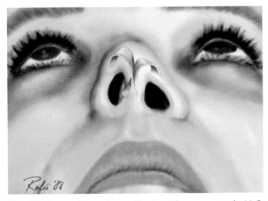

Fig. 15. Base view of a patient with asymmetric LLCs and dysmorphic nasal ala. (*From* Tollefson TT, Hum-phrey CD, Larrabee WF Jr, et al. The spectrum of iso-lated congenital nasal deformities resembling the cleft lip nasal morphology. Arch Facial Plast Surg 2011;13(3):156; with permission.)

In the alar turn-in flap technique, the cephalic portion of the LLC is transposed on a pedicle and sutured to the underside of the remaining LLC, providing additional strength to the LLC. This technique helps to support and flatten the preexisting alar concavity.

In situations in which there is significant concav-ity of the alar rim, the flip-flop technique can be used. The lateral crura of the LLC is completely dissected off the underlying vestibular skin and excised. It is then turned over, and resecured to the vestibular lining using sutures. The shape of the alar rim is then changed from concave to convex, allowing better contouring of the alar rims.

Techniques can also be combined with the use of suture repositioning and cartilage grafting. Sus-pension sutures repositioning the LLC to the upper lateral cartilage and nasal dorsum in a more super-omedial position can be used to provide better symmetry, strengthening the scroll and lateral crura.[54] In cleft rhinoplasty, these techniques are used to support and reposition the malformed alar rim cartilage.

Alar Base

In cleft lip deformity, there is asymmetry of the alar base caused by poor support of the skeletal nasal base as well as any prior surgery done before sec-ondary rhinoplasty. Malpositioning of the alar-facial junction or the insertion of the lateral alar rim is often the result of prior cleft lip repair. As a child grows, minor malpositioning during the orig-inal repair can result in a larger discrepancy and repositioning of the alar-facial junction is needed to achieve alar base symmetry.

An incomplete closure of the nasal sill is another common secondary deformity that can arise following original cleft lip repair. This deformity can be obvious if the superior portion of the orbi-cularis oris muscle is not completely closed. As a result, there is asymmetry of the alar base at the nasal sill. To an observer, there is an obvious ab-normality in the shape of the inferior aspect of the nostril. To correct this deformity, the superior aspect of the lip must be reopened to realign the underlying muscle. Furthermore, to enhance nasal base symmetry, a dermal flap or free graft can be added. In cases of minimal nasal sill deficiency, autologous fat grafting or injectable fillers can be used as an alternative.

SUMMARY

In patients with congenital cleft lip deformity, the nose is often one of the most apparent defects noted on examination. The degree of secondary nasal deformity is based on the extent of the

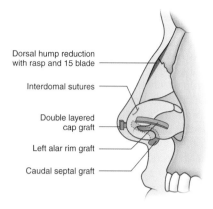

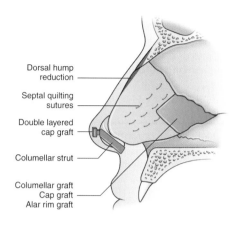

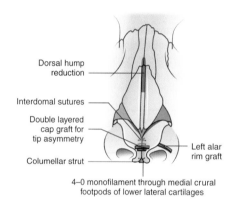

4–0 monofilament through medial crural
footpods of lower lateral cartilages

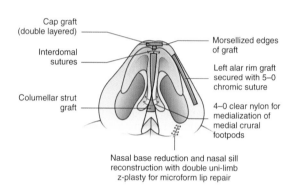

Nasal base reduction and nasal sill
reconstruction with double uni-limb
z-plasty for microform lip repair

Fig. 16. Surgical planning showing various techniques used in a definitive cleft septorhinoplasty case.

original cleft deformity, growth over time, and any prior surgical correction to the nose or lip. Repair and reconstruction of these deformities require a good understanding of the underlying pathologic anatomy, adequate surgical field exposure, and special attention to structural grafting to provide adequate support and overcome scarring. Graft material from the nasal septum, the rib, and/or the ear is often required for successful correction of these deformities. Often, it is necessary to use a combination of various techniques for the best outcome (**Fig. 16**). It is important to take into consideration both function and appearance when performing these techniques.

REFERENCES

1. Murray JC. Gene/environment causes of cleft lip and/or palate. Clin Genet 2002;61(4):248–56.
2. Wyszynski DF, Beaty TH, Maestri NE. Genetics of nonsyndromic oral clefts revisited. Cleft Palate Craniofac J 1996;33(5):406–17.
3. Tollefson TT, Shaye D, Durbin-Johnson B, et al. Cleft lip-cleft palate in Zimbabwe: estimating the distribution of the surgical burden of disease using geographic information systems. Laryngoscope 2015;125(Suppl 1):S1–14.
4. Murray JC, Schutte BC. Cleft palate: players, pathways, and pursuits. J Clin Invest 2004;113(12):1676–8.
5. Chu EA, Farrag TY, Ishii LE, et al. Threshold of visual perception of facial asymmetry in a facial paralysis model. Arch Facial Plast Surg 2011;13(1):14–9.
6. Van loon B, Maal TJ, Plooij JM, et al. 3D Stereophotogrammetric assessment of pre- and postoperative volumetric changes in the cleft lip and palate nose. Int J Oral Maxillofac Surg 2010;39(6):534–40.
7. Tollefson TT, Senders CW. Bilateral cleft lip. In: Goudy S, Tollefson TT, editors. Complete cleft care. New York: Thieme; 2015. p. 63–85.
8. Gong SG. Cranial neural crest: migratory cell behavior and regulatory networks. Exp Cell Res 2014;325(2):90–5.
9. Tollefson TT, Sykes JM. Unilateral cleft lip. In: Goudy S, Tollefson TT, editors. Complete cleft care. New York: Thieme; 2015. p. 37–62.
10. Tollefson TT, Humphrey CD, Larrabee WF Jr, et al. The spectrum of isolated congenital nasal deformities

resembling the cleft lip nasal morphology. Arch Facial Plast Surg 2011;13(3):152–60.

11. Cuzalina A, Jung C. Rhinoplasty for the cleft lip and palate patient. Oral Maxillofac Surg Clin North Am 2016;28(2):189–202.

12. Blair VP. Nasal deformities associated with congenital cleft of the lip. JAMA 1925;84:185–7.

13. McComb HK, Coghlan BA. Primary repair of the unilateral cleft lip nose: completion of a longitudinal study. Cleft Palate Craniofac J 1996;33:23–31.

14. Huffman WC, Lierle DM. Studies on the pathologic anatomy of the unilateral hare-lip nose. Plast Reconstr Surg 1949;4:225–34.

15. Avery JK. The nasal capsule in cleft palate. Anat Anz 1962;109(Suppl):722.

16. Coleman J, Sykes J. Cleft lip rhinoplasty. In: Papel ID, editor. Facial plastic and reconstructive surgery. 3rd edition. Stuttgart (NY): Thieme; 2009. p. 1082.

17. Mulliken JB. Correction of the bilateral cleft lip nasal deformity: evolution of a surgical concept. Cleft Palate Craniofac J 1992;29(6):540–5.

18. Noordhoff MS. Bilateral cleft lip reconstruction. Plast Reconstr Surg 1986;78(1):45–54.

19. Stenstrom SJ. The alar cartilage and the nasal deformity in unilateral cleft lip. Plast Reconstr Surg 1966; 38:223–31.

20. McNeil C. Orthodontic procedures in the treatment of congenital cleft palate. Dent Rec 1950;72:126–32.

21. Georgiade N, Mladick R, Thorne F. Positioning of the premaxilla in bilateral cleft lips by oral pinning and traction. Plast Reconstr Surg 1968;41:240–3.

22. Georgiade N, Latham R. Maxillary arch alignment in bilateral cleft lip and palate infant, using the pinned coaxial screw appliance. Plast Reconstr Surg 1975; 56:52–60.

23. Millard D, Latham R. Improved primary surgical and dental treatment of clefts. Plast Reconstr Surg 1990; 86:856–71.

24. Latham R. Orthodontic advancement of the cleft maxillary segment: a preliminary report. Cleft Palate J 1980;17:227–33.

25. Grayson B, Cutting C, Wood R. Preoperative columella lengthening in bilateral cleft lip and palate. Plast Reconstr Surg 1993;92:1422–3.

26. Grayson B, Cutting C. Presurgical nasoalveolar orthopedic molding in primary correction of the nose, lip, and alveolus of infants born with unilateral and bilateral clefts. Cleft Palate Craniofac J 2001;35: 193–8.

27. Singh G, Moxham B, Langley M, et al. Changes in the composition of glycosaminoglycans during normal palatogenesis in the rat. Arch Oral Biol 1994;39:401–7.

28. Matsuo K, Hirose T. Preoperative nonsurgical overcorrection of cleft lip nasal deformity. Br J Plast Surg 1991;44:5–11.

29. Matsuo K, Hirose T, Tomono T, et al. Nonsurgical correction of congenital auricular deformities in the early neonate: a preliminary report. Plast Reconstr Surg 1984;73(1):38–51.

30. Garfinkle JS, Kapadia H. Presurgical treatment. In: Goudy S, Tollefson TT, editors. Complete cleft care. New York: Thieme; 2015. p. 10–20.

31. de Ladeira PR, Alonso N. Protocols in cleft lip and palate treatment: systematic review. Plast Surg Int 2012;2012:562892.

32. Uzel A, Alparslan ZN. Long-term effects of presurgical infant orthopedics in patients with cleft lip and palate: a systematic review. Cleft Palate Craniofac J 2011;48(5):587–95.

33. Liou E, Subramanian M, Chen P, et al. The progressive changes of nasal symmetry and growth after nasoalveolar molding: a three-year follow-up study. Plast Reconstr Surg 2004;114: 858–64.

34. Pai B, Ko E, Huang C, et al. Symmetry of the nose after presurgical nasoalveolar molding in infants with unilateral cleft lip and palate: a preliminary study. Cleft Palate Craniofac J 2005;42: 658–63.

35. Abbott MM, Meara JG. Nasoalveolar molding in cleft care: is it efficacious? Plast Reconstr Surg 2012 Sep;130(3):659–66.

36. Tollefson TT, Senders CW, Sykes JM. Changing perspectives in cleft lip and palate: from acrylic to allele. Arch Facial Plast Surg 2008;10(6): 395–400.

37. Aminpour S, Tollefson TT. Recent advances in presurgical molding in cleft lip and palate. Curr Opin Otolaryngol Head Neck Surg 2008;16(4): 339–46.

38. Bennum R, Perandones C, Sepliasrsky V, et al. Nonsurgical correction of nasal deformity in unilateral complete cleft lip: a 6-year follow-up. Plast Reconstr Surg 1999;104:616–30.

39. Mulliken JB. Primary repair of bilateral cleft lip and nasal deformity. Plast Reconstr Surg 2001;108: 181–94. examination 195.

40. Mulliken JB. Repair of bilateral complete cleft lip and nasal deformity: state of the art. Cleft Palate Craniofac J 2000;37:342–7.

41. Chen PKT, Noordhoff MS. Bilateral cleft lip and nose repair. In: Losee JE, Kirschner RE, editors. Comprehensive cleft care. New York: McGraw-Hill; 2009. p. 331–342.6.

42. Yeow VKL, Chen PKT, Chen YR, et al. The use of nasal splints in the primary management of unilateral cleft nasal deformity. Plast Reconstr Surg 1999;103:1347–54.

43. Angelos P, Wang T. Revision of the cleft lip nose. Facial Plast Surg 2012;28(4):447–53.

44. Posnick JC, Thompson B. Modification of the maxillary Le Fort I osteotomy in cleft-orthognathic

surgery: the bilateral cleft lip and palate deformity. J Oral Maxillofac Surg 1993;51(1):2–11.

45. Converse JM. Corrective surgery of the nasal tip. Laryngoscope 1957;67(1):16–65.

46. Jablon JH, Sykes JM. Nasal airway problems in the cleft lip population. Facial Plast Surg Clin North AM 1999;7:391–403.

47. Haack J, Papel ID. Caudal septal deviation. Otolaryngol Clin North Am 2009;42(3):427–36.

48. Most SP. Anterior septal reconstruction: outcomes after a modified extracorporeal septoplasty technique. Arch Facial Plast Surg 2006;8(3):202–7.

49. Cutting C. Cleft lip nasal reconstruction. In: Rees TD, LaTrenta GS, editors. Aesthetic plastic surgery. Philadelphia: Saunders; 1994. p. 497–532.

50. Guryuron B. MOC-PS(SM) CME article: late cleft lip nasal deformity. Plast Reconstr Surg 2008;121(4, Suppl):1–11.

51. Kridel RW, Scott BA, Foda HM. The tongue-in-groove technique in septorhinoplasty. A 10-year experience. Arch Facial Plast Surg 1999;1(4):246–56.

52. Shih CW, Sykes JM. Correction of the cleft-lip nasal deformity. Facial Plast Surg 2002;18(4):253–62.

53. Murakami CS, Barrera JE, Most SP. Preserving structural integrity of the alar cartilage in aesthetic rhinoplasty using a cephalic turn-in flap. Arch Facial Plast Surg 2009;11(2):126–8.

54. Tajima S, Maruyama M. Reverse-U incision for secondary repair of cleft lip nose. Plast Reconstr Surg 1977;60(2):256–61.

The Saddle Deformity
Camouflage and Reconstruction

CrossMark

Jon Robitschek, MD[a],*, Peter Hilger, MD, FACS[b]

KEYWORDS

- Saddle nose deformity • Nasal dorsal reconstruction • Allograft materials

KEY POINTS

- This article presents a comprehensive review of past and present modalities in the surgical management of saddle nose deformities.
- Various surgical techniques, including allograft materials, are systematically reviewed.
- The senior author's (Hilger P) surgical experience and current management approach are highlighted.

INTRODUCTION

The saddle nose deformity constitutes one the most exacting anatomic, functional, and aesthetic challenges encountered by nasal reconstructive surgeons. Success dictates an approach focused on an understanding of the presenting etiology, precise anatomic analysis, and comprehensive surgical planning. Within a surgeon's armamentarium, there has evolved a wide breadth of surgical options to effectively camouflage and reconstruct the saddle nose deformity. Operative management strives to achieve critical success in addressing the external aesthetic deformity and the inherent loss of functional nasal integrity. What follows is an in-depth review of these basic tenets in the operative intervention for the saddle nose deformity as well as the salient features in their technical execution.

ETIOLOGY AND DIAGNOSTIC CONSIDERATIONS

The principal anatomic deformity in the saddle deformity revolves around a deficit in nasal dorsal support secondary to the loss of septal cartilage and/or nasal bone height (**Fig. 1**). The presenting etiology can be divided into 3 basic categories:

iatrogenic, traumatic injury, and medical disease. Prior to the advent of nasal surgery, infectious causes, including septal abscess, syphilis, and leprosy, were the predominate disease entities.[1] In the modern surgical era, operative sequela and traumatic injury constitute the vast majority of today's saddle nose cases.

A minority of cases can, however, be linked to medical conditions whose nasal manifestations exhibit erosion of the dorsal septal cartilage and often degradation of other structural elements as well as crucial changes in the internal and external epithelial envelope. A differential diagnosis, including cocaine abuse, intranasal malignancy, and systemic inflammatory disease, warrant preoperative consideration.[2] This latter group encompasses relapsing polychondritis, Crohn disease,[3] sarcoidosis,[4] lupus erythematous, and Wegener granulomatosis.[5] In the vast majority of cases, a thorough screening history and focused physical examination, including anterior rhinoscopy, is sufficient to exclude an occult disease process. Resolution or, at minimum, stabilization of the metabolic disorders must be sought before surgical considerations.

Select patients with mucosal ulcerations, history of chronic sinusitis, or septal perforation can be considered for further investigation. Additional

Disclosure Statement: The authors have nothing to disclose.
[a] University of Minnesota, 7373 France Avenue Suite #410, Edina, MN 55435, USA; [b] Facial Plastic & Reconstructive Surgery, University of Minnesota, 7373 France Avenue Suite #410, Edina, MN 55435, USA
* Corresponding author.
E-mail address: robitschekjm@gmail.com

Facial Plast Surg Clin N Am 25 (2017) 239–250
http://dx.doi.org/10.1016/j.fsc.2016.12.007
1064-7406/17/Published by Elsevier Inc.

facialplastic.theclinics.com

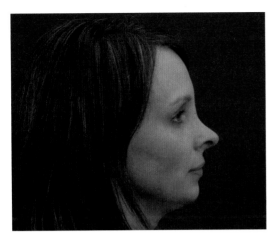

Fig. 1. Patient with a moderate to severe saddle nose deformity.

diagnostic modalities include nasal endoscopy, septal biopsy, and screening sinus CT scan or chest radiograph. Laboratory assessment in select cases includes erythrocyte sedimentation rate (ESR), C-reactive protein (CRP), angiotensin-converting enzyme (ACE), fluorescent treponemal antibody absorption, and antineutrophilic cytoplasmic antibodies (ANCAs). As to how extensive preoperative work-up should be, the sensitivity and overall clinical utility of nasal biopsies in cases of septal perforations and nasal ulcers are limited.[6] Of the laboratory tests, ANCAs and ACE are more helpful than CRP and ESR in elucidating a systemic process among those patients with intranasal findings.[7] Again, relying on a focused clinical history and physical examination more often than not excludes these rare entities. If chemical dependence is the genesis of the deformity, then prolonged sobriety must be the primary goal before surgical intervention. The authors have found the soft tissue contraction and vascular compromise provoked by cocaine abuse extremely challenging.

The clinical history should focus on prior nasal surgeries, trauma exposure, and nasal symptoms. For patients with a past history of nasal surgery and/or trauma, reviewing prior operation reports and CT imaging as well as preinjury photographs can be beneficial in gauging anatomic deficits, characterizing the premorbid state, and constructing a successful reconstruction sequence. Focused inquiry on symptoms of nasal obstruction enable both the surgeon and the patient to engage on the intricate link between form and function. From the perspective of both parties, it is especially important to delineate dynamic from fixed obstruction, anatomic from reactive pathology, and surgical benchmarks from medical management. As with any clinical endeavor with cosmetic implications, a patient's sense of self and

individual perception of the ideal nasal anesthetic assume center stage in the development of a successful treatment plan. Such success is born from a thorough clinical history during the initial consultation.

PHYSICAL EXAMINATION AND CLASSIFICATION

The foundation of precise surgical management originates with a thorough physical examination, including both internal and external nasal components.[8] Manual palpation of the nasal subunits yields significant information with regard to structural tip support, pliability of soft tissues, length of nasal bones, premaxillary support, and skin characteristics. Performing a Cottle maneuver, including its modified version, aids in establishing the role of the external and internal valve in nasal obstruction.[9] It is helpful to evaluate the health of the nasal mucosa because some diseases demonstrate metaplasia of the respiratory epithelium with squamous cell replacement and resultant dry crusted debris accumulation. Decongestion of the nasal mucosa in the clinic permits delineation of dynamic obstruction and facilitates a complete examination of the nasal septum. As a principal dorsal support mechanism and a key contributor in the saddle presentation, the nasal septum with its associated mechanical strength, structural integrity, and contour needs to be fully assessed. Rhinomanometry and acoustic rhinometry represent useful adjuncts in quantifying nasal patency and may offer some predictive value in gauging surgical benefit with septoplasty alone when coupled with the physical examination. Rhinoscopy, cotton swab palpation, and nasal endoscopy constitute the primary tools for the surgeon in defining the contributions of the nasal septum to both dorsal and tip support as well as functional obstruction.[10,11]

One of the core concepts in nasal reconstruction is evaluation of the skin soft tissue envelope (SSTE). As a fixed resource, the SSTE often serves as the limiting factor in how aggressive structural adjuncts might be placed into the nose. Housing the nasal bony and cartilaginous scaffold, the SSTE includes both the internal mucosal lining and the external skin. Manual palpation of the nasal tip and dorsum with digital manipulation of the internal nasal vestibule provides insight into skin tension, points of contracture, and pliability of the cartilage interface. Avenues to expand the SSTE may include skin grafting as well as local or composite grafting. Failure to incorporate the SSTE component in the reconstruction template, particularly in cases of revision surgery and prior trauma, frustrates the overall outcome.[12]

In terms of stratifying the saddle nose deformity, there are several anatomic classification schemes in the literature. Integrating elements of progressive bony and cartilaginous deficits, these classifications systems can be helpful in establishing a rational approach to surgical intervention.[13,14] One such system, offered by Daniel and Brenner in 2006,[15] outlines a spectrum of saddle deformities ranging from mild depression of the dorsal cartilage to significant collapse of the bony vault (**Fig. 2**). Because each individual nose may be funneled into a specific category, an anatomic centered approach in ascribing the severity of the nasal deformity has considerable merit. Accepting the premise that every nose is unique, the authors further submit that a tiered, structure-based evaluation aids surgeons in determining the right operation for the right nose. Focusing on the septum as the principal support mechanism provides surgeons a foundation to reconstitute dorsal projection, tip posture, and bony contour (**Fig. 3**). Integrating these fundamental concepts with the preoperative physical examination and photographic analysis supplies the framework for precise surgical planning.

PATIENT COUNSELING

With respect to preoperative counseling, only 14% of what is shared in verbal communication likely is retained.[16] The skeletal and soft tissue distortions seen with these deformities require that patient and surgeon have a realistic image of what can be achieved with surgical intervention. Successful surgical outcomes for the saddle nose deformity often require more than 1 operation, with a reported minor revision rate ranging from 11% to 30%.[17] Accepting the inherent variability in graft resorption, stable construct positioning, limited SSTE elasticity, and possible warping, it is important to educate patients on the complexity of the task at hand. It is the practice of the senior author to actively engage patients in a shared long-term perspective on achieving an optimal outcome. Moreover, in the authors' experience, secondary surgical refinements are beneficial for approximately 30% of these patients.[18] These should be candidly discussed with patients prior to the consideration of any surgery so that all involved in a patient's care appreciate the complexity of these cases and refinement surgery. Combating the myopic view of a singular intervention with immediate permanency, patient counseling incorporates a frank conversation on the role and indications for minor revisions. This is understood to be part of the global care plan rather than a surgical failure of the initial operative plan. Even in the

best of circumstances, the ultimate outcome is a compromise from the ideal and such expectations are essential if patient and surgeon are to be pleased. It is of particular import in cases of revision surgery, contracted SSTE, and bony vault reconstructions, where more than 1 consultation may be indicated. Establishing shared expectations between surgeon and patient is essential in moving forward from the day of surgery to when the cast comes off and, perhaps most importantly, the 12-month follow-up.

SURGICAL MANAGEMENT

The efforts of Weir and Roe in late nineteenth-century New York state highlight the genesis of modern-day rhinoplasty.[19,20] Valiant attempts to address the saddle deformity have incorporated a broad range of graft material ranging from ivory to gold to even the occasional sternum of a recently deceased duck (**Fig. 4**).[21] The grasp of nasal anatomy has matured in step with an empirical understanding of the limits in nasal augmentation material. Today's reconstructive surgeons avail themselves of several options, including transient camouflage, autologous grafting, alloplastic implants, and homograft material. The fundamental challenge, however, remains not so much which material is used but rather the when, where, and rationale of how it is used. Assimilating the preoperative examination and the occasional intraoperative revelation, the reconstructive surgeon's approach should incorporate an expectation and willingness to alter the surgical plan intraoperatively.

Referencing the tiered structural evaluation (see **Fig. 3**), surgical management is tailored to a 3-pronged graduated approach. Functional collapse of the dorsum is often associated with sacrifice of vertical nasal length, tip malposition, and a recessed columella. Stabilization and reinforcement of septal support serve as the foundation for correct tip positioning and dorsal augmentation. Progressively building support into these anatomically interdependent structures serves to enable contour augmentation and counteracts the inherent contractive forces of the SSTE (**Fig. 5**) while correcting the airway impairment.

The nasal septum represents the cornerstone of dorsal support and needs to be formally addressed in surgical planning. Prior to focusing on the essential elements of tip posture and dorsal augmentation, the strength and mechanical support of the septum should be optimized. If there is a perforation amendable to repair, consideration for primary closure can be entertained in a combined or, rarely, a staged procedure. If the septum

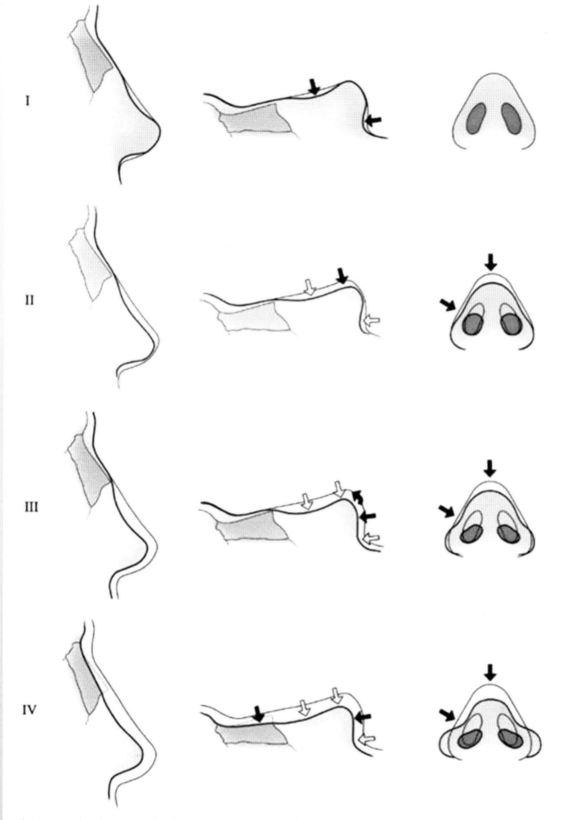

Fig. 2. Daniel and Brenner classification scheme. Progressive range beginning with type I demonstrating intact septal support with mild supratip depression and columellar retrusion. Type IV – complete collapse of bony and cartlaginous vault, shortened columella and tip over rotation. Arrows represent vectors of soft tissue and bony contracture. Type II and III represent progressive degrees of soft tissue loss and structural collapse. (*From* Daniel RK, Brenner KA. Saddle nose deformity: a new classification and treatment. Facial Plast Surg Clin North Am 2006;14(4):304; with permission.)

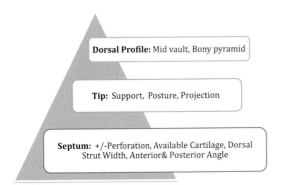

Dorsal Profile: Mid vault, Bony pyramid

Tip: Support, Posture, Projection

Septum: +/-Perforation, Available Cartilage, Dorsal Strut Width, Anterior& Posterior Angle

Fig. 3. Tiered preoperative structural assessment.

is intact, there is often a clear deficiency in the width or the height of the dorsal strut and caudal strut, respectively. The traditional septal L-strut of a 1.5-cm dorsal and caudal scaffold serves as a useful blueprint in the traditional nose, but the saddle nose is often depleted of septal resources and replete with structural laxity and scar. Addressing the septum in full, whether complete reconstruction with cartilage grafts, establishing a foundation in the premaxilla, or reinforcement with septal struts, sets the stage for subsequent tip and dorsal refinement. The premaxilla is an often overlooked concept and a significant contributor to the retraction seen at the colu-mellar-labial angle (**Fig. 6**).

With a reinforced nasal septum serving as the foundation, attention can be focused on establish-ing correct tip posture, shape, and projection. As the dorsum loses projection in the typical saddle presentation, the nasal tip demonstrates cephalad rotation with associated loss of domal support and projection. This effective shortening of the nasal length is partially addressed with septal optimiza-tion (see **Fig. 5**), but the tip support mechanics need to be formally addressed. In classifying various interventions to the tip apparatus, a useful

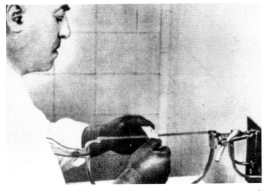

Fig. 4. Dr Jacques Joseph carving an ivory exograft nasal graft (circa 1918).

construct involves delineating adjuncts that directly influence the nasal vestibule versus the SSTE. For example, a caudal septal extension graft, tip onlay grafts, or caudal strut can demon-strably influence tip projection whereas a lateral crural strut stabilizes the external valve. Additional considerations include the position and contour of the premaxilla, which assumes an integral role in contextualizing the ideal tip posture. Lastly, extended spreader grafts offer another option for influencing the internal valve and stabilization of the tip. The distensibility of the nasal lining is usu-ally the limiting factor as structural grafts are added to increase the projection of the lower half of the nose, derotate the tip, and correct columella and ala contours and proportions. Expending the nasal lining with composite grafts and or local flaps, such as a turbinate flap, as discussed later, may be required to accommodate the additional structure in the surgical plan. If the airway is adequate and only a limited amount of projection or derotation is sought, then onlay grafts can enhance the external nasal dimensions without further increase in the internal cross-sectional area (**Fig. 7**).

Having established a dorsal septal platform with stable tip position, dorsal augmentation is the denouement of the reconstruction. Deciding on the appropriate material, harvest site consider-ations, and appropriate preoperative counseling is a significant step prior to arriving at this final phase of the reconstruction. The technique and material composition of dorsal augmentation in the saddle nose is widely variable in the litera-ture[17,22] (**Fig. 8**). The critical elements in dorsal augmentation typically revolve around the ques-tions of how much is needed, where to place it, and what material is going to be used. A funda-mental query must be answered prior to augmen-tation: Is the objective to correct the external nasal contour exclusively or does the deformity mandate expansion of the of the internal nasal dimension with associated physiologic improvement?

If the latter situation is a goal of the surgical plan, then the dorsal augmentation should be con-structed as an onlay spreader graft. This approach enlarges the intranasal space by widening the nasal valve, and traction of the dorsal volume addi-tion on the nasal side walls further expands the airway and adds stiffness. This circumstance precludes the use of alloplastic material and, in the authors' opinion, is best accomplished with autologous structure. Mirroring a graduated clas-sification scheme and a progressive operative blueprint, mild cases might only require a low pro-file onlay graft to the midvault. On the opposite end of the spectrum, more severe cases might only be

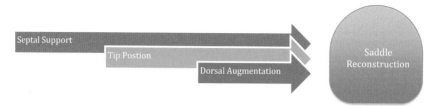

Fig. 5. Graduated stepwise approach to reconstruction of the saddle nose.

successfully addressed with a dorsal spanning osseocartilaginous composite graft.

Allograft Dorsal Correction

The advantages of alloplastic implants include their availability, ease in shaping, and avoidance of donor site complications. Disadvantages include risks of implant extrusion, infection, and displacement. Implant placement benefits from a generous soft tissue barrier from mucosa to protect against contamination from the nasal cavity. In the modern surgical era, the principal 3 materials used in dorsal augmentation are high-density porous polyethylene (HDPP) (Medpor [STRYKER Corporation, Kalamazoo, MI, USA]), expanded polytetraflouroethylene (e-PTFE), and silicone.

HDPP implant consists of interconnected pores (125–250 μm) with a malleable semirigid texture. Promoting soft tissue ingrowth and neovascularization, HDPP offers a stable material with minimal risk of long-term resorption. e-PTFE demonstrates similar characteristics with a pore size of 10 μm to 30 μm and limited superficial soft tissue ingrowth. A comparative advantage of e-PTFE rests with its softer contour compared with the stiffness of HDPP.[23] As to risk of infection for HDPP and e-PTFE, several groups having reported rates between 3.2% and 10.7%. Similarly, rates of implant extrusion are slightly higher, ranging from 3.2% to 16.1%.[24]

In Asia, silicone implants have garnered wide appeal with supportive evidence of their long-term efficacy.[25] Forming a fibrous capsule without tissue ingrowth, silicone offers an easily carved platform for dorsal augmentation. Micromotion of the implant itself can potentiate displacement and extrusion. Speaking to the success in the Asian patient population, a thick SSTE seems to provide a protective buffer for implant longevity. The reported relative rates of infection and extrusion are comparable to e-PTFE and HDPP[26] (**Table 1**).

Homograft Dorsal Correction

Ranging from cadaveric bone and rib grafts to acellular dermis, homograft dorsal augmentation offers an alternative to allograft implants (**Figs. 9 and 10**). Yielding a lower rate of extrusion and infection compared with allograft material, cadaveric rib and bone offer the distinct advantages of availability and no donor site morbidity. The authors find homograft rib cartilage acceptable for smaller deformities when limited contraction pressure is applied to the graft. Downsides include rigid texture and contour in cases of bone and the risk of resorption and warping with rib cartilage and bone. Comparative studies between irradiated homograft rib and autologous ribs grafts have not demonstrated a clear advantage for cartilage grafts with regard to resorption, infection, and warping.[27]

Acellular dermis (AlloDerm [ALLERGAN, Irvine, CA, USA]) has been used to provide modest augmentation to the dorsum with low rates of infection, seroma formation, and extrusion. Combining AlloDerm with diced cartilage for dorsal augmentation has been reported as a useful construct in saddle nose reconstruction.[28] Highly compliant and offering a soft contour, AlloDerm's principal detractors when used exclusively remain its limited volume and gradual significant resorption over time and thus the authors do not use it for these cases.[29]

Autologous Dorsal Correction

Adhering to the tenet of replacing like with like, autologous grafting of the dorsum remains the

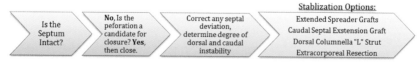

Fig. 6. Optimizing the septum's integrity, contour, and mechanical strength.

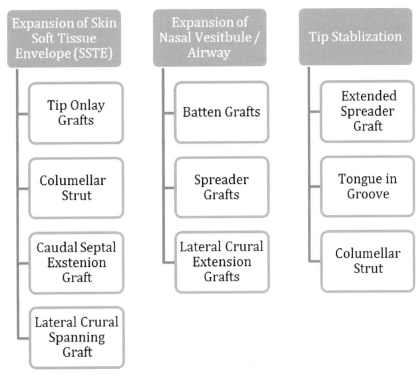

Fig. 7. Establishing tip contour, posture, and projection.

historical gold standard in saddle nose reconstruction and is the authors' preferred augmentation resource. Compared with allograft implants, the reported rates of infection, displacement, and extrusion for autologous grafts are lower. When weighing autologous versus homologous cartilage grafts, here is little evidence to convincingly state that one is considerably superior to the other.

Septal cartilage is the most common source of graft material in a majority of rhinoplasty cases; however, in saddle nose reconstruction it is often absent, insufficient in volume, or woefully deficient. Auricular cartilage is easy to harvest, with minimal donor site morbidity. Potential disadvantages to auricular cartilage include its curved contour and relative thin structure compared with septal cartilage. Dicing harvested cartilage into 2-mm to 3-mm fragments and using temporalis fascia, AlloDerm, or tissue glue affords an alternative to monolayer or laminated onlay grafts. Diced cartilage augmentation strives to maximize the volume of dorsal projection with a fixed amount

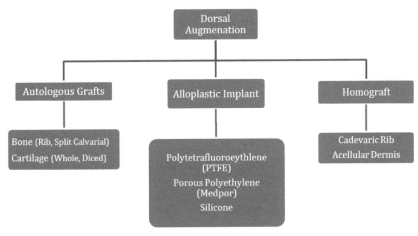

Fig. 8. Avenues of dorsal augmentation.

Table 1
Comparison of Allopastic implants for dorsal augmentation

Material	Pros	Cons
Silicone	Capsule formation, ease of removal, soft contour	No vascular ingrowth, extrusion, infection
High-density porous polyethylene (Medpor)	Significant vascular ingrowth, malleable	Difficult to remove, extrusion, rigid texture, infection
Expanded-polytetrafluoroeythlene (Gore-Tex [GORE Medical Products, Flagstaff, AZ, USA])	Moderate vascular ingrowth, soft contour	Extrusion, infection displacement

of cartilage availability. Diced cartilage is a reasonable option for a moderate saddle nose and has been a tool for the nasal reconstructive surgeon since the 1940s.[30] It is appropriate when contour enhancement is the surgical goal and expansion of the nasal airway is not required (**Fig. 11**).

The severity and anatomic composition of dorsal depression dictate the volume, texture, and quantity of grafting material. When the deformity involves collapse of the bony pyramid and severe posterior displacement of the midvault, the capability of septal or auricular onlay grafts is often exceeded. In such cases, attention is typically directed toward autologous bone and cartilage rib, including split calvarial and osseocartilaginous composite grafts. The benefits of such graft material include its strength and relative abundance compared with septal or auricular sources. The comparative disadvantages include donor site morbidity, warping, surgical time, and texture mismatch.

Split calvarial bone grafts offer considerable structure support but have limited capacity for contouring and leave the nose with a rigid texture. Autologous rib cartilage is generally considered the gold standard in saddle nose reconstruction and can be harvested exclusively or as a composite osseocartilaginous construct. The advantages of autologous rib rests with its abundance, ability to be contoured, and comparatively low rate of resorption over time. The donor site morbidity for rib harvest is one of its greatest detractors with complications, including pneumothorax, hematoma, scar, prolonged postoperative recovery, and infection. The literature reports a combined risk of donor site complication as less than 3%, with hypertrophic chest scarring the most common. Other disadvantages include warping and displacement with reported rates of 3% and 0.5%, respectively.[31]

Risk of gradual warping of rib cartilage is a genuine concern and has prompted considerable discussion in the literature. Preventive strategies include concentric carving, allowing the cartilage to soak for 15 to 30 minutes in 0.9% saline, suture fixation, concentric lamination, and accordion-style scoring cuts.[17] Despite such measures, delayed warping or graft displacement can be incredibly vexing for surgeon and patient. Such frustrations have led the senior author to explore other avenues for managing severe saddle deformities.

The composite osseocartilaginous graft is a unique hybrid construct with several benefits, including limited risk of warping, and is the authors' preferred resource for structural support in moderate to severe deformities. The reconstruction is performed through an open rhinoplasty approach with the upper lateral cartilages separated from the nasal septum. The graft is harvested from the tenth floating rib and is of sufficient length to cover the entire dorsal unit. Compared with harvesting a strictly cartilaginous graft from ribs 6 to 8, the bony cartilaginous junction must be preserved with at least 3 cm to 5 cm of incorporated bone. Risk of fracture at this stress junction can be reduced by freeing the medial portion of cartilage entirely from its perichondrial sleeve prior to making the lateral bone cut. A 4-mm cutting bur is used to precisely contour the graft, creating a hollowed-out ventral depression for the bony dorsum and nasal septum. The cartilaginous portion of the final construct is generally 25% to 30% of the entire dorsal length. The cephalald portion of the onlay is tapered to diminish the risk of a palpable lateral overhang.

The osseocartilaginous graft allows bone-to-bone contact with the bony pyramid, which facilitates osseous integration. A critical element to promoting osseous integration of the graft centers on adequate preparation of the bony edifice on which it rests. Lateral osteotomies are performed when necessary to widen the bony base. This is followed by gently burring down the bony dorsum with a 4-mm cutting bur to establish a freshened and level platform on which the graft rests. To create the ideal dorsal profile, the graft spans the entire nasal length from the radix to the interdomal region. Next, the upper lateral cartilages are sutured to the caudal lateral portions of the graft

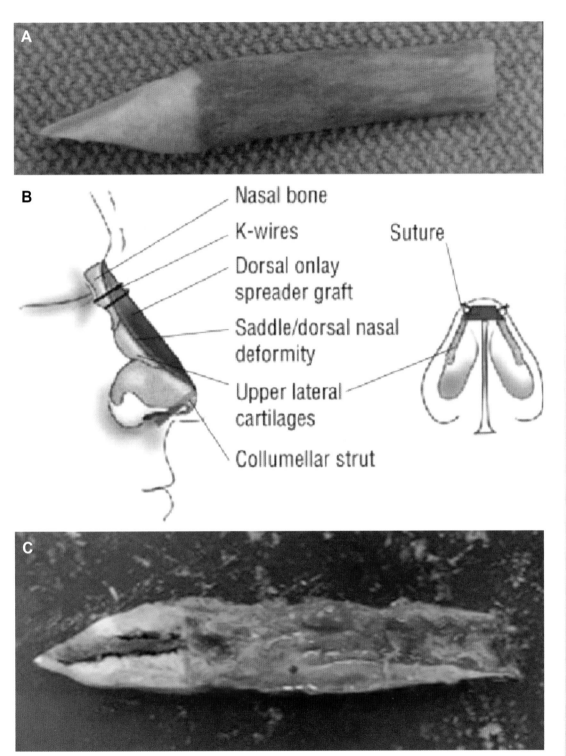

Fig. 9. Autologous osseocartlaginous rib graft reconstruction. (*A*) Dorsal aspect of graft. (*B*) Structural outline of graft placement. (*C*) Ventral aspect of graft.

through either cartilage or predrilled holes. This maneuver, in effect, creates an onlay spreader graft, which expands the internal nasal valve and widens the midvault profile (**Table 2**).

There are several options to combat displacement of graft material. Suture fixation to the lower lateral cartilages, as described previously, is helpful, but 2-point fixation is ideal. Using 2 threaded

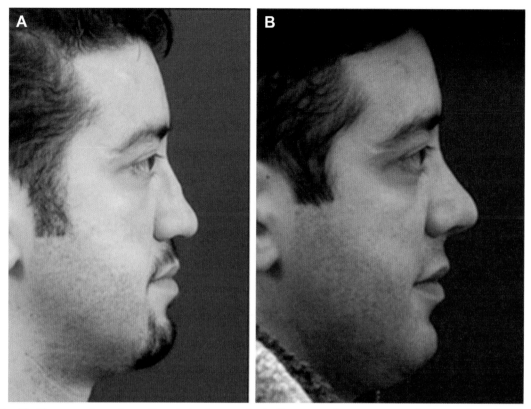

Fig. 10. Three-month postoperative photos from patient after an autologous osseocartilaginous rib graft reconstruction. (A) Preoperative photo. (B) Postoperative photo.

0.035-in threaded Kirschner wires through the dorsum provided excellent graft stabilization. A typical nasal cast in placed over the wires and they are generally removed in clinic without difficulty in 3 weeks. Other options include titanium screw fixation, horizontal wiring, and cephalic suture placement. Whichever technique is used, stabilization of the onlay graft is helpful in promoting tissue integration and preventing displacement.

SURGICAL ADJUNCTS AND PEARLS

Using a multifaceted approach, several adjuncts the authors have found useful include a generous columella strut and a premaxillary cartilage graft in the context of a recessed nasolabial angle. In an effort to stabilize the columnella strut, the authors create a shallow V niche in the anterior maxillary spine using a 2-mm osteotome with figure-of-eight suture (5-0 polydioxanone) fixation to the periosteum. Additionally, the authors find nasal sidewall support in the low half of the nose an essential component to improving the nasal airway. In the authors' reported experience, the most common need for revision centered on recurrent nasal obstruction that was subsequently addressed with batten, lateral crural strut, or endonasal spreader graft placement.[19]

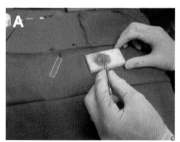 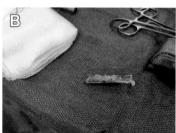 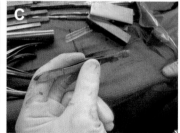

Fig. 11. (A) Diced (2–3 mm fragments) cartilage dorsal onlay graft. Created using TISSEEL fibrin sealant and a bivalved 3-mL syringe (B, C).

Table 2
Comparison of autologous and homograft materials

Material	Pros	Cons
Acellular dermis (AlloDerm)	Readily available, ease of placement, soft contour	High resorption rate, limited volume
Homograft rib cartilage graft	No donor site morbidity, availability	Warping, infection, extrusion, brittle
Septal cartilage graft	Easy to harvest and contour, low infection/extrusion rate	Often unavailable in revision cases, limited volume
Auricular cartilage graft	Low donor site mobility, low risk of infection/extrusion	Curved contour, limited amount, thin
Diced cartilage graft	Maximizes a fixed cartilage resource	Resorption, limited volume
Split calvarial bone graft	Rigid structural support	Donor site morbidity, unable to contour, firm feel to the nose
Autologous cartilaginous rib graft	Gold standard for cases of severe saddle nose deformity	Donor site morbidity, infection, resorption, warping
Autologous osseocartilaginous rib graft	Bone-to-bone contact, replaced like with like	Donor site morbidity, infection, resorption, warping

A contracted nasal lining is a complex challenge when contemplating projection, denotation, and expansion of the airway. Beyond the tools discussed previously, the authors have found success with composite cartilage grafts to the nasal vestibule and local mucosal flaps from the inferior turbinate, particularly in the context of adhesions and vestibular stenosis. In rare but extreme cases of lower-third contraction, the surgeon may need to use techniques usually reserved for oncologic reconstruction, such as forehead flap resurfacing of the nasal tip. This is usually performed hand in hand with a variety of lining reconstruction techniques that are beyond the scope of this discussion.

REVISION CASES

The revision rate of saddle nose reconstruction is considered higher than in primary rhinoplasty cases. Reported complication rates with subsequent revision are widely variable depending on technique used, surgeon's experience, severity of the presenting deformity, and how "complication" is defined. Three themes have characterized the senior author's approach over the past 3 decades. First, it is essential that surgeon and patient engage in a thorough preoperative counseling on the patient's expectations. Second, it is important that the plan not be timid but uses an aggressive approach. Such a strategy incorporates major structural grafts compared with more limited tactics using smaller grafts that provide some camouflage but fail to address the full scope of the

deformity. Finally, all parties must understand the complexities of the problem and appreciate that secondary intervention should not be viewed as failure of the surgical endeavor but enhancement that addresses the frequent outcome variations that can be expected in complex wounds.

CONCLUDING THOUGHTS

The surgical management of saddle nose reconstruction can be equally challenging, vexing, and satisfying. The defect harbors both functional and aesthetic manifestations, with surgical correction drawing on all facets of corrective nasal surgery. A sound diagnostic approach and thorough preoperative counseling set the stage for surgical success. Beginning with the reinforcement of the nasal septum and tip posture, the authors advocate a progressive reconstructive approach. Dorsal augmentation is an essential component, but the structural framework on which it rests is core.

Each dorsal graft material has its own unique profile that can vary among patient populations and surgeon preference. What may work well in the hands of one group may not easily translate to another. The authors' particular approach favors autologous grafting when available and, in particular, finds the osseocartilaginous graft a boon in moderate to severe cases. With limited warping potential and the capacity for bone-to-bone integration, the composite osseocartilaginous construct is a useful tool to augment the entire dorsum, from radix to tip.

REFERENCES

1. Daniel RK. Rhinoplasty: septal saddle nose deformity and composite reconstruction. Plast Reconstr Surg 2007;119:1029–43.
2. Guerrero MT, Cárdenas-Camarena L, Rodríguez-Carrillo J. Nasal angiocentric lymphoma: an entity that should be remembered. Ann Plast Surg 2001; 46(2):178–82.
3. Merkonidis C, Verma S, Salam MA. Saddle nose deformity in a patient with Crohn's disease. J Laryngol Otol 2005;119(7):573–6.
4. Baum ED. Sarcoidosis with nasal obstruction and septal perforation. Ear Nose Throat J 1998;77: 896–902.
5. Schreiber BE, Twigg S, Keat AC. Saddle-nose deformities in the rheumatology clinic. Ear Nose Throat J 2014;93(4–5):E45–7.
6. Murray A, McGarry GW. The clinical value of septal perforation biopsy. Clin Otolaryngol Allied Sci 2000;25(2):107–9.
7. Diamantopoulos II, Jones NS. The investigation of nasal septal perforations and ulcers. J Laryngol Otol 2001;115(7):541–4.
8. Alsarraf R, Murakami CS. The saddle nose deformity. Facial Plast Surg Clin North Am 1999;7:303–10.
9. Fung E, Hong P, Moore C, et al. The effectiveness of modified cottle maneuver in predicting outcomes in functional rhinoplasty. Plast Surg Int 2014;2014: 618313.
10. Haavisto LE, Sipilä JI. Acoustic rhinometry, rhinomanometry and visual analogue scale before and after septal surgery: a prospective 10-year follow-up. Clin Otolaryngol 2013;38(1):23–9.
11. Pirilä T, Tikanto J. Acoustic rhinometry and rhinomanometry in the preoperative screening of septal surgery patients. Am J Rhinol Allergy 2009;23(6): 605–9.
12. Kim DW, Toriumi DM. Management of posttraumatic nasal deformities: the crooked nose and the saddle nose. Facial Plast Surg Clin North Am 2004;12(1): 111–32.
13. Emsen IM. New and detailed classification of saddle nose deformities: step-by-step surgical approach using the current techniques for each group. Aesthetic Plast Surg 2008;32(2):274–85.
14. Pribitkin EA, Ezzat WH. Classification and treatment of the saddle nose deformity. Otolaryngol Clin North Am 2009;42(3):437–61.
15. Daniel RK, Brenner KA. Saddle nose deformity: a new classification and treatment. Facial Plast Surg Clin North Am 2006;14(4):301–12.
16. Kessels RP. Patients' memory for medical information. J R Soc Med 2003;96(5):219–22.

17. Ozturan O, Aksoy F, Veyseller B. Severe saddle nose: choices for augmentation and application of accordion technique against warping. Aesthetic Plast Surg 2013;37:106–16.
18. Christophel JJ, Hilger PA. Osseocartilaginous rib graft Rhinoplasty: a stable, predictable technique for major dorsal reconstruction. Arch Facial Plast Surg 2011;13(2):78–83.
19. Roe JO. The deformity termed "Pug-Nose" and its correction, by a simple operation. Arch Otolaryngol Head Neck Surg 1989;115(2):156–7.
20. Weir RF. On restoring sunken noses without scarring the face. 1892. Aesthetic Plast Surg 1988; 12(4):203–6.
21. Lupo G. The history of aesthetic rhinoplasty: special emphasis on the saddle nose. Aesthetic Plast Surg 1997;21(5):309–27.
22. Romo T, Sclafani AP. Reconstruction of the major saddle nose deformity using composite allo-implants. Facial Plast Surg 1998;14(2):151–7.
23. Ferril GR, Wudel JM, Winkler AA. Management of complications from alloplastic implants in rhinoplasty. Curr Opin Otolaryngol Head Neck Surg 2013;21(4):372–8.
24. Wang TD. Multicenter evaluation of subcutaneous augmentation material implants. Arch Facial Plast Surg 2003;5(2):153–4.
25. Tham C, Lai YL, Weng CJ. Silicone augmentation rhinoplasty in an Oriental population. Ann Plast Surg 2005;54:1–5.
26. Colton JJ, Beekhuis GJ. Use of Mersilene mesh in nasal augmentation. Facial Plast Surg 1992;8(3): 149–56.
27. Kridel RW, Ashoori F, Hart CG. Long-term use and follow-up of irradiated homologous costal cartilage grafts in the nose. Arch Facial Plast Surg 2009; 11(6):378–94.
28. Gordon CR, Habal MB, Papay F. Diced cartilage grafts wrapped in AlloDerm for dorsal nasal augmentation. J Craniofac Surg 2011;22(4):1196–9.
29. Sherris DA, Oriel BS. Human acellular dermal matrix grafts for rhinoplasty. Aesthet Surg J 2011; 31(7):95–100.
30. Tasman AJ, Diener PA, Litschel R. The diced cartilage glue graft for nasal augmentation morphometric evidence of longevity. JAMA Facial Plast Surg 2013;15(2):86–94.
31. Wee JH, Park MH, Jin HR. Complications associated with autologous rib cartilage use in rhinoplasty: a meta-analysis. JAMA Facial Plast Surg 2015;17(1): 49–55.

Revision Functional Surgery: Salvaging Function

Sahar Nadimi, MD[a,b], David W. Kim, MD[c,d],*

KEYWORDS

- Revision rhinoplasty • Functional rhinoplasty • Nasal valve • Rhinoplasty complications

KEY POINTS

- A smooth, symmetric, well-proportioned surface contour with a stable underlying structural foundation is the ultimate aesthetic goal for rhinoplasty.
- The relationship between the upper and lower lateral cartilages and the septum is crucial in maintaining nasal tip and dorsal support.
- Secondary nasal obstruction is commonly caused by inward malposition of the upper lateral cartilages and internal valve area and/or collapse of the lateral crura and external valve incurred during reductive primary surgery.
- Correction of middle vault collapse may be accomplished through spreader grafts that may be extended in a cephalic, caudal, or dorsal direction depending on anatomic need.
- Correction of lateral wall collapse is effectively treated with lateral crural strut grafts (LCSGs), which may have variable length, stiffness, and position depending on degree of pathology.

INTRODUCTION

Rhinoplasty has been described as one of the most challenging procedures in plastic surgery, with revision rates reported as high as 15% to 20% after primary procedures.[1,2] Many rhinoplasty techniques rely on resection of the nasal osseocartilaginous framework to achieve aesthetic objectives. The weakened nasal framework remaining after reductive surgery may have inadequate strength to withstand the contractile forces of healing.[3,4] Patients often present with significant aesthetic and functional deformities requiring revision surgery.

The unfavorable interplay of soft tissue contracture and a weakened structural framework can lead to severe obstruction and cosmetic deformity. In revision rhinoplasty, the surgeon may need to build new constructs out of transplanted material that mimics the shape and function of the original anatomy. Thus, when revision rhinoplasty aims to rebuild a nose that has been over-reduced and structurally compromised, the task is incredibly difficult.

There are several categories of rhinoplasty complication (**Table 1**). In cases of postrhinoplasty nasal obstruction, the most likely causes are destabilization of nasal structures and/or excessive reduction or excision of the nasal framework. The most common areas in which these problems occur are in the middle vault and lateral walls of the nose. In the middle vault, cartilaginous hump reduction, especially when accompanied by narrowing osteotomies, leads to inferomedial

a Department of Otolaryngology, Head and Neck Surgery, Loyola University Medical Center, 2160 South First Avenue, Maywood, IL 60153, USA; b Private Practice, Facial Plastic and Reconstructive Surgery, 1S 280 Summit, Suite C-4, Oakbrook Terrace, IL 60181, USA; c Division of Facial Plastic and Reconstructive Surgery, Department of Otolaryngology–Head and Neck Surgery, University of California, San Francisco, 55 Francisco Street, Suite 705, San Francisco, CA 94103, USA; d Private Practice, Facial Plastic and Reconstructive Surgery, 55 Francisco Street, Suite 705, San Francisco, CA 94133, USA
* Corresponding author. Division of Facial Plastic and Reconstructive Surgery, Department of Otolaryngology–Head and Neck Surgery, University of California, San Francisco, 55 Francisco Street, Suite 705, San Francisco, CA 94103.
E-mail address: dwk@drkimfacialplastics.com

Facial Plast Surg Clin N Am 25 (2017) 251–262
http://dx.doi.org/10.1016/j.fsc.2016.12.008

Table 1
Common rhinoplasty errors

Minor (error of technique)	• Asymmetric structural modification (eg, bone cut or cartilage sutures) • Malpositioned cartilage graft • Malpositioned implant	• Asymmetric nose • Palpable or visible graft • Palpable or visible implant (possible infection)
Error of omission (failure to execute a needed step)	• Various	• Persistent original problem (eg, persistent dorsal hump, twisted nose, asymmetric middle vault, and various tip deformities)
Failure to restabilize structures that have been weakened during surgery	• Failure to stabilize nasal base • Failure to stabilize the nasal bridge • Failure to stabilize outer wall	• Drooping nasal tip • Pinched nose (bridge), internal nasal obstruction. • Pinching of the nasal tip, nasal obstruction
Excessive excision (overaggressive reduction of the nose)	• Lower edge of the septum • Nasal tip cartilages • Nasal bridge • Nostril base	• Short nose, upturned nose, retracted columella • Tip irregularity, tip collapse, nasal obstruction • Scooped dorsum, ski-sloped nose, nasal obstruction • Overly narrow nostrils, slitlike nostrils, nasal obstruction
Gross error of judgment	• Various	• Possible severe deformity

migration of the upper lateral cartilages and internal valve compromise. In the lower nose, narrowing tip techniques lead to medialization of the lateral crura and alar and external valve collapse.

Correction of these deformities is best treated with structural grafting techniques that strengthen the compromised anatomic structures and restore their stable relationships to one another.

PREOPERATIVE ASSESSMENT

The consultation between a patient seeking a revision rhinoplasty and a surgeon is crucial to understanding motivations and establishing common goals. The magnitude of functional impairment should be determined. Utilization of the Nasal Obstruction Symptom Evaluation (NOSE) instrument can help quantify the degree of obstruction and also track improvement and long-term function after revision.[5] Patients must understand that revision surgery is more difficult, with potentially limited outcomes given the degree of trauma incurred previously. Patients with previous reduction rhinoplasty and functional impairment should understand that certain areas of the nose may need to be expanded to allow for restored function. Use of digital imaging to render such visual outcomes may be helpful in these cases. Surgery should only be undertaken

if both patient and surgeon have reached common and realistic goals.

When evaluating the revision rhinoplasty patient, it is important to determine what surgery has been done in the past, along with the timing and number of previous procedures. Old operative notes are sometimes helpful but should never be taken at face value, because they may not contain all details of the previous procedure. The external nasal contour and the internal airway must be assessed to diagnose and localize the deformities.

An accurate assessment of the aesthetic and functional problems helps surgeons formulate a surgical plan and select the appropriate techniques.

The physical examination should be conducted in a systemic fashion. The symmetry and width of the nose should be assessed on frontal view, including evaluation of the brow-tip aesthetic line, which can help to identify middle vault deformities, such as middle vault collapse or an inverted-V deformity. These features may reveal an underlying middle vault and internal valve compromise. Assessment of the lower third of the nose is important to assess lateral wall stability and contour. Findings, such as dynamic inspiratory collapse, alar retraction, supra-alar pinching, alar narrowing, and bossae, may be evidence of previous destructive tip work. Both inspection and palpation of the nasal septum should be performed to determine abundance, stability, and position of the nasal septum.

MIDDLE VAULT

In normal nasal anatomy, the middle vault consists of the paired upper lateral cartilages and their associated internal nasal mucosa. The upper lateral cartilages support the internal valve and determine the external contour of the middle third of the nose. The upper lateral cartilages attach cephalically with the nasal bones and medially with the cartilaginous septum. At their upper aspect, the upper lateral cartilages display a dome-shaped cross-sectional geometry, conforming the shape of the nasal bones as they emerge from the undersurface of the bones. Here, the upper lateral cartilages fuse to one another horizontally across the dorsum. Caudally, the upper lateral cartilages take on a more triangular cross-sectional geometry. In this region, they are associated with the paired lower lateral cartilages forming the scroll region. The internal nasal valve area is defined as the connection between the caudal margin of the upper lateral cartilage, the head of the inferior turbinate, the floor of the nose, and the septum. Often in an unoperated nose, this is naturally the narrowest point of airflow and area of greatest flow resistance.

The most common obstructive problem seen in the middle vault in revision rhinoplasty is malposition of the upper lateral cartilages in a medial, inferior, and/or ventral direction. This is often due to collapse of the upper lateral cartilage onto the dorsal septum after cartilaginous hump reduction, especially when the dorsal margin of the upper lateral cartilages is resected en bloc with the dorsal margin of the septum. This maneuver greatly reduces the dorsal-ventral dimension of the upper lateral cartilages, leading to the characteristic inferomedial malposition along with the associated middle vault pinching, characterized by deep vertical shadows flanking the dorsum. These problems may also involve an inverted-V deformity in which the caudal aspect of the nasal bones are skeletonized and visibly revealed due to the upper lateral cartilages pulling away from the bones inward. The three-fourths view is particularly helpful in assessing middle vault and internal valve 3-D deficiency, because the upper lateral cartilage depression is seen as a contour depression from this oblique angle. Patients with short nasal bones and long upper lateral cartilages are especially prone to these problems. Aggressive narrowing osteotomies can exacerbate the above middle vault problems by causing additional medialization

of the upper lateral cartilages, by virtue of their connection to the nasal bones.

There are several strategies that may be used to prevent these problems during primary rhinoplasty. First, the amount of hump reduction may be minimized by preserving dorsal height. Adding radix volume and/or increasing tip projection in certain cases may allow for less dorsal reduction while still resulting in a straighter dorsum. Second, preserving the dorsal-ventral length of the upper lateral cartilages may reduce the risk of inward collapse of the upper lateral cartilages after hump reduction. This requires that component reduction of the hump be performed, in which the upper lateral cartilages are first separated from the dorsal septum and the septum lowered first. Preserving upper lateral cartilage dorsal height may then allow for inward folding of the upper lateral cartilages (spreader flap or autospreader) to maintain middle vault stability and function. Third, spreader grafts can be used to restore or precisely modulate middle vault and internal valve width and support.

In cases of revision surgery for the over-reduced nose, the spreader grafting technique is most helpful. There is usually a deficiency of native upper lateral cartilage left for in-folding and the dorsal septum has been overly lowered. It is the preference of the senior author (Kim DW) to approach this correction through an open rhinoplasty approach with an anterior dissection to the dorsal septum, typically first by establishing a submucoperichondrial plane at the anterior septal angle. This dissection must be executed meticulously because prior caudal septal truncation and septal harvest may have distorted the anatomic landmarks and tissue planes. If a weak, compromised L-strut is encountered, a decision must be made as to whether or not the L-strut is strong enough to serve as a foundation for the subsequent spreader grafts (and, if needed, tip work). If L-strut reconstruction is needed, this should be done at this point prior to any work on the middle vault or tip.[6]

At this point, the surgeon must determine the appropriate dimensions of the spreader grafts. The frontal width should be assessed by using both internal and external landmarks. Internally, the cephalic aspect of the spreader grafts should be wide enough to provide a smooth transition to bony dorsal aesthetic line. Ideally, the graft allows for a smooth transition between the bony vault in 3-D. This is best checked by assessing continuity with the skin envelope down after spreader graft placement from several perspectives (frontal, lateral, and all angles between). If there is asymmetry of the dorsal septum, asymmetric width of the spreader grafts can help camouflage this.

Caudally, the spreader graft width should taper as it approaches the anterior septal angle but remain wide enough to support and open the internal valve. In many cases, multiple layered spreader grafts may be needed to provide enough width for any given revision nose (**Fig. 1**).

The cephalic-caudal length of the classic spreader graft spans along the cephalic-caudal length of the exposed upper lateral cartilage. In the revision nose, however, the spreader graft may need to be longer than usual, extending cephalically, caudally, or in both directions. Cephalic extension may be indicated to fill in the contour depression of a bony open roof, particularly if the bony base is too narrow to allow for medializing osteotomies. Additionally, cephalically extended spreader graft may be useful to splint nasal bones laterally after out-fracture for the over-narrow bony vault. Caudal extension of the spreader graft may be needed to support a septal extension graft or septal replacement graft (**Fig. 2**). When long spreader grafts are needed, multiple graft may be needed, placed end to end with one another.

The dorsal-ventral dimension of a spreader graft should be at minimum 3 mm to 4 mm. This length is needed to ensure stability and long-term integration to the dorsal septum. In some cases in which the dorsal septum has been overly lowered, the spreader graft may be made to be taller (greater dorsal-ventral dimension) so that it extends dorsally above the existing dorsal septum. This is useful for some saddle deformities, in which the septal height is compromised but the upper lateral cartilages are intact and have adequate dorsal length to stretch articulate with the new dorsal spreader graft margin. This may help correct collapse of the upper lateral cartilages in these situations, opening the internal valve area. If there is a deficiency of upper lateral cartilage from prior resection, there may be limitation of dorsal migration of the upper lateral cartilages limiting the dorsal extension of the spreader graft. In these cases, an additional onlay graft over the middle vault reconstruction may be necessary to optimize dorsal height.

The material for the grafts should come from autologous cartilage. Septal cartilage is ideal,

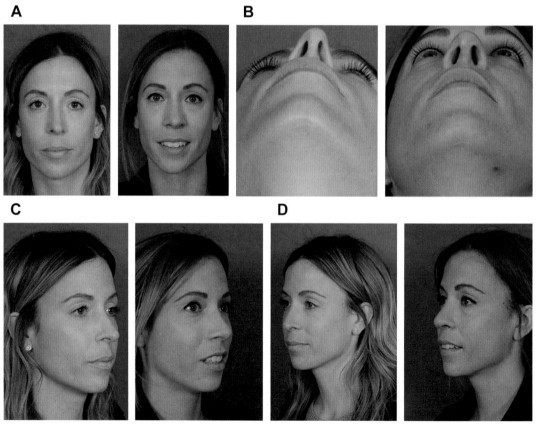

Fig. 1. Patient with asymmetric collapse of middle vault and internal valves. Double-thickness spreader grafts 403 were used on her right side and single thickness on her left side. Preoperative (*left*) and postoperative (*right*) views. (*A*) frontal, (*B*) base, (*C*) left three-fourths, and (*D*) right three-fourths.

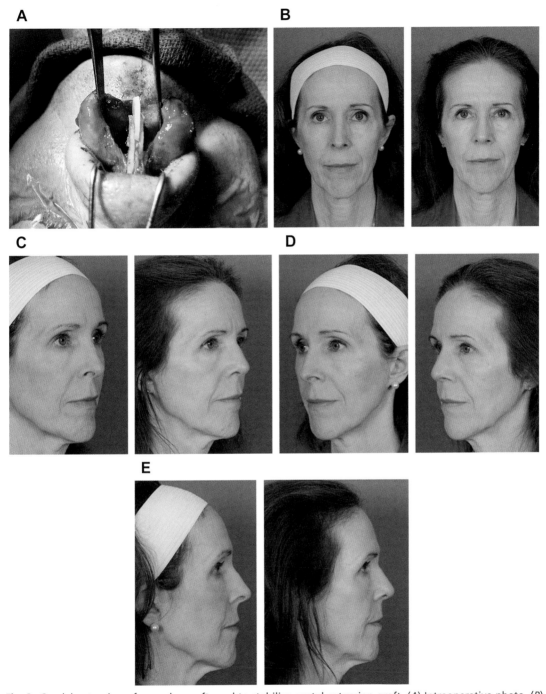

Fig. 2. Caudal extension of spreader graft used to stabilize septal extension graft. (*A*) Intraoperative photo. (*B*) Preoperative (*left*) and postoperative (*right*) frontal photos of patient with middle vault and internal valve collapse as well as a crooked caudal septum. Long spreader grafts were placed to correct her internal valve issues as well as to stabilize a midline septal extension graft. (*C*) Right three-fourths view, (*D*) left three-fourths view, and (*E*) right lateral view.

although there may not be available septum in the revision nose due to prior resection. Either auricular cartilage or costal cartilage may be used for spreader grafts. Because auricular cartilage is curved, the surgeon must account for this when placing grafts. For example, orienting grafts with opposite curvatures on each side of the nose can lead to on overall straight contour. When spreader grafts need bear structural load (caudal or dorsal extension, for example), costal cartilage is preferred by virtue of greater stiffness and strength. When costal cartilage is used, the grafts should be carved from the center of the specimen to reduce the tendency for warping.[7]

Once the grafts are created, they should be inserted between the dorsal margin of the upper lateral cartilages and dorsal septum (or desired dorsal line in cases of dorsal extension). It is the preference of the senior author to use several 5-0 polydioxanone suture (PDS, Ethicon) horizontal mattress sutures for fixation. These fixation sutures may be placed on a slight bias to tension the caudal aspect of the L-strut toward one side (helpful for a crooked L-strut). This maneuver, known as the clocking suture, uses an angled mattress suture with the fixation more cephalic one on side and more caudal on the other. The caudal L-strut complex then moves slightly toward the side with the cephalic fixation.

NASAL TIP/LATERAL WALL

The nasal tip is comprised of the C-shaped lower lateral cartilages that can be subclassified as medial, intermediate, and lateral crura. The inherent stiffness and length of the lower lateral cartilages, their connection to the upper lateral cartilages in the scroll areas, and the support to the lower lateral cartilage from the caudal septum make up the major mechanisms of tip support. The

contour and position of the lateral crura spanning from dome to posterior termination help support the nostril margin and external valve. The lateral crural surface contour also determines variations of tip shape. When the lateral crura are convex the tip tends to be bulbous and wide. When the lateral crura are concave, the tip is pinched, isolated laterally by deep shadows, or ball-shaped.

The wide variations in the lower lateral cartilage contour accounts for the massive diversity of nasal tip shape. Excessive tip prominence is often perceived as undesirable and is, therefore, a common motivation for rhinoplasty. The reflexive treatment of some surgeons is to make the tip narrower or smaller, sometimes at the cost of stability or function. Techniques that attempt to reduce bulk or bulbosity through excision, to narrow through division of the lower lateral cartilage intact strip, or to cinch in the domal contours through aggressive suture methods all tend to create a gathering and bunching of tip cartilages into the midline at the cost of weakness, medialization, and collapse laterally. This results in external valve compromise with inspiratory collapse as well as an unattractive, pinched, overdone-appearing nasal tip (**Fig. 3**).

These problems can be lessened in primary rhinoplasty if a surgeon adheres to certain principles. The goal should be to create changes in shape rather than simply creating reduction in size and width. A soft triangular base of the nose is optimal for appearance and function, with relative

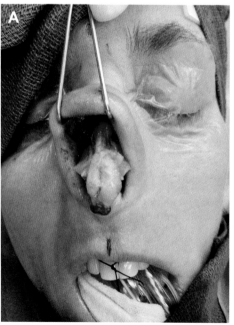
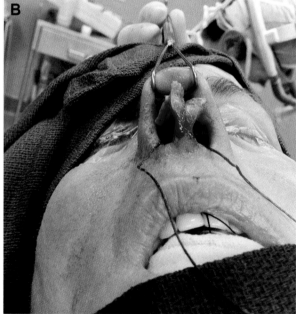

Fig. 3. Intraoperative photos of over-resected lateral crura. (*A*) Frontal view. (*B*) Base view.

narrowness at the domes, relative width at the alar base, and an unbroken straight or slightly convex transition between the 2 is ideal.[8] The lateral crura must be stable and smooth along their length for this to be present. Conservative suture and excision techniques may be sufficient as long as they do not compromise structural integrity. When greater changes are needed, structural grafting techniques may be a better option. The senior author uses a combination of a septal extension graft, tongue-in-groove stabilization of the lower lateral cartilages, LCSGs, and suture modulation in more than 50% of primary rhinoplasty to precisely control contour and function. When these structural principles are followed, significant aesthetic gain can be attained without compromising function. This has be corroborated in a recent prospective multicenter cohort study by the senior author, in which nasal obstruction symptoms were evaluated in aesthetic-functional rhinoplasties performed. Nasal symptoms were evaluated using the NOSE scale. The 2 major methods for nasal valve reconstruction used were spreader grafts and alar-batten grafts, both of which were found effective in treating patients with nasal valve insufficiency. Aesthetic interventions were stratified into tip interventions (dome suture, lateral crus cephalic trim, lateral crus strut, and tip repositioning) and vault interventions (hump reduction, dorsum augmentation, and osteotomies). Both the functional and aesthetic-functional groups had a similar magnitude of improvement in nasal breathing, with mean improvements in the NOSE scale score of 51 and 47 at 3-month assessments, respectively. Thus, combining aesthetic interventions with functional rhinoplasty does not seem to alter the magnitude of improvement in nasal breathing outcome.[9]

In the revision of functionally impaired nose, the lateral crura are often compromised through prior excessive excision, scoring or morselization, or aggressive narrowing, resulting in alar collapse and lateral wall/external valve insufficiency. The senior author prefers to address these deformities through structural grafting techniques performed through an external rhinoplasty approach. The same combination of steps is used as in many primary rhinoplasties (septal extension graft, tongue-in-groove stabilization, LCSGs, and suture stabilization), but the techniques must be adjusted for the degree of damage to be corrected.

A prerequisite to lateral wall reconstruction is first establishing midline stabilization of the tip tripod complex. The senior author prefers to use a strong septal extension graft as the basis of this stabilization. In revision surgery, the graft must often bear a greater load than in primary surgery because the position of the tip may need to be greatly altered (as in the case of the foreshortened nose or droopy tip).

The general steps for the septal extension graft and tongue-in-groove stabilization is as follows:

1. Establish a stable caudal structure for which tip tripod can be secured via a septal extension graft or a septal replacement graft depending on the L-strut. This graft must be strong enough to leverage the associated load. For example if the nose needs to be lengthened, the graft must be long, strong, and stable enough to push the tip complex down and forward into a stiff soft tissue covering. Side-to-side fixation with multiple suture points can be used, typically with 5-0 PDS mattress sutures. End-to-end fixation is an alternative and has the advantage of using less cartilage and incurring less width in the columella and caudal septum. The smaller surface area of contact between the native caudal septum and in-line septal extension graft means it requires additional stabilizing maneuver to provide sufficient strength. For example, the graft may be designed to be long, abutting the nasal spine and suture stabilized through a transverse drill hole at the base of the nasal spine. Several additional points of fixation to the existing caudal septum with thin splinting grafts that flank the articulation of the caudal septum and the extension graft are also typically performed. Fixation to the caudal aspects of the extended spreader grafts, which project beyond the native anterior septal angle, also provide a powerful mechanism of stabilization. The authors use a combination of 5-0 clear nylon and PDS sutures for these areas of fixation. The goal is for the caudal graft to be stable and midline (**Fig. 4**).

2. Next, a tongue-in-groove fixation of the medial and intermediate crura is set to the desired tip projection and rotation. In many cases of revision surgery, the nose is short and there are soft tissue constraints that prevent the tip and domes from reaching the optimal position. Wide dissection of the entire soft tissue covering and using long marginal incisions gain some mobility of the tip tripod. If the desired projection and rotation are reached, the surgery can then move on to addressing tip shape issues.

3. If the tripod is still over-rotated and/or underprojected at this point due to limited mobility of the tripod, the lateral crura may need to be dissected completely free from the underlying vestibular lining, reinforced with a backing extended LCSG (eLCSG), and stabilized into a

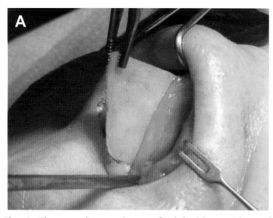 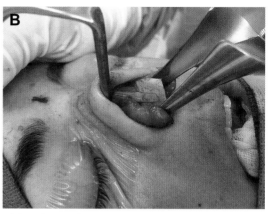

Fig. 4. The septal extension graft. (*A*) Side-to-side graft. (*B*) End-to-end graft stabilized by extended spreader grafts.

lateral, low pocket into the alar lobule. This maneuver frees the lateral crura from their soft tissue attachments and provides more mobility to the tripod. In the method, the medial extent of the LCSG can be adjusted to alter the position of the dome of the lower lateral cartilage, moving it more medially to deproject the nose (medial crural steal) or more laterally to increase projection (lateral crural steal). If the tip is significantly projected or counter-rotated with this approach, there may be deficiency of internal lining to accommodate the expanded tripod and extensive vestibular undermining may be needed to allow for closure. Rarely, a composite graft may need to be inserted into the marginal incision to provide more lining. This method is discussed in greater detail later.

Once the tip tripod is stabilized and tip position is set, the correction of the lateral wall insufficiency may be performed. If the native lateral crura are in continuity from domes to termination and have sufficient cephalic-caudal width, LCSGs are usually sufficient for treatment that allow for a natural, soft external contour. The LCSG allows for improvement of the shape and stability of the tip/ base geometry while maintaining the natural superficial location of the native lateral crura.

Although alar batten grafts are commonly cited as a work-horse technique for the treatment of lateral wall insufficiency and nasal valve problems, the senior author strongly believes this technique is inferior to the LCSG in virtually all cases. The main problems with the alar batten graft is the lack of leverage. That is, the batten graft, even if wide and outwardly convex, is not stabilized and leveraged onto stable points of fixation. Because it is an onlay graft, the alar batten graft is limited in creating lateralization of the lateral wall, with

the tendency for the graft to pull inward to the damaged or medially positioned lateral crura. To overcome this, the surgeon may be tempted to use a very large or convex graft, which then leads to cosmetic deformity. The LCSG, in contrast, is leveraged onto the fixed septal extension graft in the midline and into the dense stiff tissue at the alar lobule posteriorly. In severe cases, a long eLCSG is stabilized into a tight long pocket extending posteriorly and laterally from the end of the marginal incision into the stiff alar lobular fibrous tissue (**Fig. 5**).

Our approach to the execution of the LCSG follows a sequence of maneuvers. Once the tripod is stabilized by a tongue-in-groove approach, the authors set the dome position slightly less projected than ideal in anticipation that there generally will be 2 mm to 3 mm of additional projection from placement of the LCSGs and accompanying dome sutures. The vestibular mucosa is dissected away from the undersurface of the lateral crura from desired domal position to posterior termination, except for the caudal free edge of the lateral crura. The LCSG is then inserted beneath the lateral crura along the caudal aspect. The dimensions and shape of the LCSG vary and should be equivalent to prevent asymmetries or deviation of the tip. The anterior edge of the LCSG should be beveled to allow for an appropriate domal angle and divergence for the proper vector of the LCSG from dome to base. In most cases, the authors use longer grafts that span beyond the areas of collapse but to the termination of the lateral crura. The posterior termination of the grafts are stabilized into a snug pocket at the end of the marginal incision toward the alar base. Several 5-0 PDS horizontal mattress sutures are used to stabilize the graft to the underside of the lateral crura.

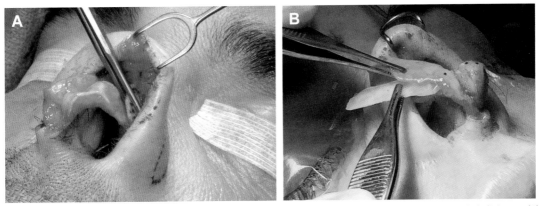

Fig. 5. (*A*) The alar batten graft is an onlay graft with limited control of correcting lateral crural deficiency. (*B*) The LCSG provides more control of lateral crural support and contour as it is leveraged medially by the septal extension graft and laterally by the firm alar lobular tissue.

Transdomal and intradomal sutures are then placed to set tip width and lateral wall contour. Placement of these sutures along the cephalic aspect of the lateral crura and domes tends to rotate the caudal aspect of the lateral crura construct anteriorly, thus increasing support to the alar margin and external valve. This can, however, create hollowing in the scroll areas, which may need to be offset with thin onlay camouflage grafting.

In cases in which the native lateral crura are malpositioned cephalically, the alar margins are retracted, or the tip overall is significantly foreshortened, the lateral crura may need to be repositioned. Here, the lateral crura are dissected completely free from the underlying epithelium (including the caudal margin), the LCSGs are placed, and the entire construct is positioned more caudally than the original location. This is accomplished through placement of eLCSGs, which are longer than traditional grafts. The termination of the eLCSGs is stabilized into a pocket with a more caudal vector, allowing for a

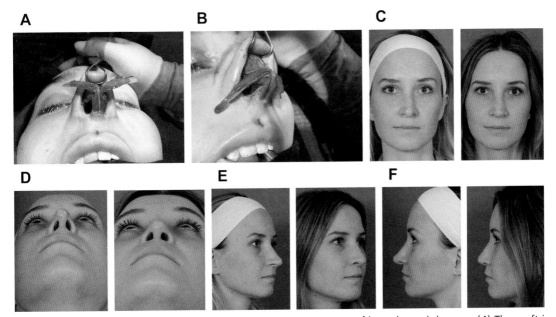

Fig. 6. The eLCSG is a powerful technique to correct even severe cases of lateral crural damage. (*A*) The graft is secured to the undersurface of the native lateral crura. (*B*) Dome sutures are placed after the graft is stabilized to set tip shape and contour. (*C*) Preoperative (*left*) and postoperative (*right*) photos of patient who received eLCSG with medial crural steal to strengthen her lateral walls/external valves as well as deproject her domes. The eLCSGs extended medial to her preoperative dome position to create a new domal angle to allow for deprojection. She also received dorsal augmentation. (*D*) Base view, (*E*) right three-fourths view, and (*F*) left lateral view.

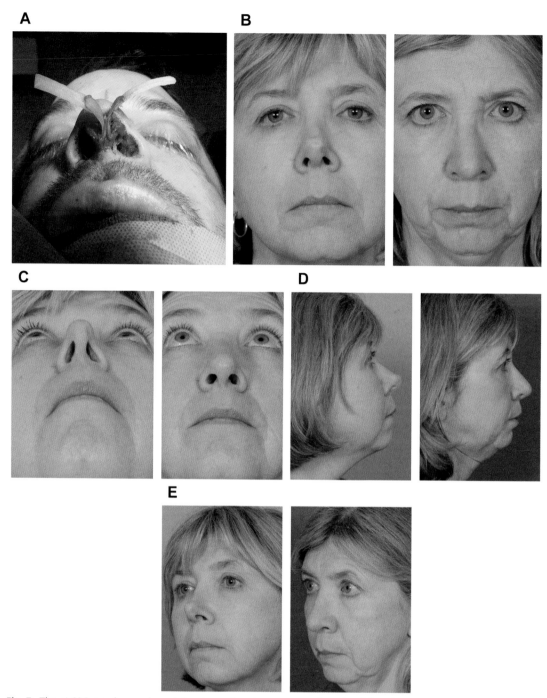

Fig. 7. The eLCSG may be used as a lateral crural replacement graft and stabilized onto a small remnant of lower lateral cartilage in the most severe cases of lateral crural resection. (*A*) Rib cartilage was used to create an eLCSG, which is anchored to a remnant of native lateral crus (anchored to the septal extension graft). (*B*) Preoperative (*left*) and postoperative (*right*) frontal vies of a patient (different from intraoperative photo) who had very aggressive resection of almost all her lateral crura. Correction with eLCSGs from costal cartilage. (*C*) Base view, (*D*) right lateral view, and (*E*) left three-fourths view.

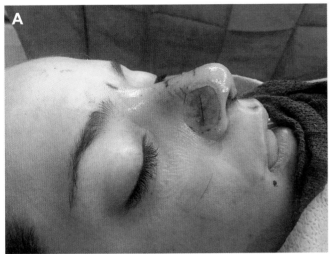
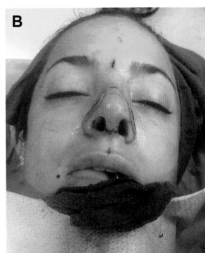

Fig. 8. (*A, B*) Transalar splints sutured in place.

mechanical downward force of the lateral wall and nostril margin. In essence, the stiff lateral crural construct leverages against 2 fixed points at its origin at the domes (stabilized by tongue in groove) and the termination is inside a snug pocket in the stiff alar soft tissue. The eLCSG may also be used to reposition the lateral crura posteriorly and thus allow for significant deprojection of the tip. In this variation, the eLCSG is positioned to extend medial to the preexisting dome bend, essentially creating a medial crural steal effect. The lateral/posterior aspect of the graft and attached lateral crura slide posteriorly into the soft tissue pocket at the alar lobule (**Fig. 6**).

In the most severe cases, there is insufficient lateral crura and a patient requires a lateral crural replacement graft. The shape and size of such grafts are similar to the eLCSG but there is little native lateral crural cartilage overlapping the graft. It is difficult to replicate this soft bend between medial crura and lateral crura with a graft, particularly when constructed from rib cartilage. If needed, a small segment of softer cartilage (excised lateral crura or cross-hatched septal cartilage) can be fixated onto the anterior aspect of the caudal septal graft and the lateral crural replacement graft can be anchored to it. The same considerations apply with the eLCSG with regard to symmetry, anterior beveling, and posterior stabilization apply. This technique is also useful when the native tip tripod is limited in the extent to which it can repositioned forward. In such cases, the tripod can be divided between the stable intermediate and medial crura and the intermediate and lateral crural component of the tripod can gain mobilization, allowing for significantly more projection (**Fig. 7**).

For all the lateral crural techniques described, the ability of the internal vestibular lining to stretch over the lateral crural construct to close the marginal incisions should not be ignored. In the presence of excised internal lining or vestibular webbing or when significant expansion or projection is needed, these incisions may not close easily. The vestibular lining is mobile to some degree through undermining more cephalically up to the level of the middle vault and upper lateral cartilages. Otherwise, composite grafts are used and the senior author obtains such grafts from an anterior approach at the cymba concha with full-thickness skin grafting of the donor site if needed. The grafts should be cut to appropriate dimension and inset circumferentially into the lining defect and then bolster stabilized for 5 days to 7 days postoperatively.

If the underlying vestibular mucosa is undermined off the lateral crura, a transalar splint is placed to ensure apposition of the lining onto the lateral crural construct. Most commonly, oval-shaped segments of a thin fluoroplastic material (0.25-mm Reuter Bivalve Fluroplastic Intranasal Splint) stabilized by a 3-0 nylon horizontal mattress suture are used. Overtightening of the suture should be avoided to prevent skin necrosis (**Fig. 8**).

SUMMARY

The information presented describes the senior surgeon's approach to treating revision rhinoplasty patients with nasal obstruction caused by weakening and structural compromise. These problems most commonly manifest in the middle vault and lateral walls of the nose. The aggressive, mainly reductive, primary rhinoplasty methods leading to these problems are still unfortunately widely used. Management requires careful analysis and thoughtful surgical planning. In the middle vault, spreader graft reconstruction is the most useful and versatile tool to restore function and 3-D contour. The spreader grafts may be extended in a cephalic, caudal, or dorsal direction, depending on need. For lateral wall and lateral crural reconstruction, the tip tripod should be stabilized onto a strong septal extension graft and then LCSGs may be used to control contour and support of the lateral crura themselves. Again, the LCSGs can be altered in length and position depending on severity of deformity. By understanding the 3-D anatomy of the middle vault and nasal base and becoming facile with structural grafting techniques, surgeons can effectively correct these difficult functional problems while creating a cosmetically favorable shape of the nose.

REFERENCES

1. Papel ID. Secondary rhinoplasty. In: Papel I, editor. Facial plastic and reconstructive surgery. 3rd edition. New York: Thieme; 2009. p. 589–603.

2. Mazzola RF, Felisati G. Secondary rhinoplasty: analysis of the deformity and guidelines for management. Facial Plast Surg 1997;13:163–77.

3. Brenner MJ, Hilger PA. Grafting in rhinoplasty. Facial Plast Surg Clin North Am 2009;17:91–113.

4. Toriumi DM. Structure approach in rhinoplasty. Facial Plast Surg Clin North Am 2002;10:1–22.

5. Stewart MG, Witsell DL, Smith TL. Development and validation of the Nasal Obstruction Symptom Evaluation (NOSE) scale. Otolaryngol Head Neck Surg 2004;130:157–63.

6. Kim DW, Gurney T. Management of nasoseptal L-strut deformities. Facial Plast Surg 2006;22:9–27.

7. Kim DW, Shah AR, Toriumi DM. Concentric and eccentric carved costal cartilage: a comparison of warping. Arch Facial Plast Surg 2006;8:42–6.

8. Toriumi DM, Checcone MA. New concepts in nasal tip contouring. Facial Plast Surg Clin N Am 2009;17:55–90.

9. Yeung A, Hassouneh B, Kim DW. Outcome of nasal valve obstruction after functional and aesthetic-functional rhinoplasty. JAMA Facial Plast Surg 2016;18:128–34.

Advances in Technology for Functional Rhinoplasty
The Next Frontier

Sachin S. Pawar, MD[a],*, Guilherme J.M. Garcia, PhD[a,b], John S. Rhee, MD, MPH[a]

KEYWORDS

- Finite element modeling (FEM) • Computational fluid dynamics (CFD) • Virtual surgery
- Computer modeling • Simulation • Nasal surgery • Rhinoplasty • Septoplasty

KEY POINTS

- Computer modeling and simulation technologies have the potential to provide facial plastic surgeons with information and tools that can aid in patient-specific surgical planning for rhinoplasty.
- Finite element modeling and computational fluid dynamics (CFD) are modeling technologies that have been applied to the nose to study structural biomechanics and nasal airflow.
- Patient-specific computational models can be modified to simulate surgical changes or perform virtual surgery. CFD tools can then be used to study the effects of these changes on nasal function and, in the future, aid in surgical planning and in predicting surgical outcomes.

INTRODUCTION

Among all of the procedures in facial plastic surgery, rhinoplasty demands the highest level of understanding in aesthetics, soft and hard tissue dynamics, and the delicate interplay between form and function. Adding to the complexity of this procedure are individual patient factors that can impact patient outcomes, including variable anatomy and medical comorbidities. The techniques currently used have evolved through many years of hard work, ingenuity, and experimentation of numerous rhinoplasty surgeons. Collectively, this comprises decades of knowledge that has largely been developed through individual surgeon experience and, undoubtedly, trial and error.

Advances in computer-based modeling and simulation are now providing ways to better study and understand individual anatomy, tissue dynamics, and specific surgical techniques. Modeling has been used in engineering fields for decades

and has helped engineers design complex processes and products for numerous industries. Methods for finite element modeling (FEM) and computational fluid dynamics (CFD) were first introduced in the 1950s and 1960s, and limited to applications within various engineering fields. As computing technology has advanced, applications for modeling and simulation have slowly expanded to medicine and, more recently, applied to nasal anatomy and rhinoplasty techniques.

Surgical modeling is not an entirely new concept. Craniofacial surgeons have been performing model surgery for decades, using cephalometric measurements and physical resin molds to plan and design orthognathic surgery and facial skeletal dimensions preoperatively.[1] Using model surgery, they could make better informed decisions about the specific maneuvers needed to achieve the desired outcome for a patient, specific to that patient's anatomy and clinical requirements. In short, this type of model surgery minimizes the

[a] Department of Otolaryngology and Communication Sciences, Medical College of Wisconsin, 9200 West Wisconsin Avenue, Milwaukee, WI 53226, USA; [b] Department of Biomedical Engineering, Marquette University & the Medical College of Wisconsin, 9200 West Wisconsin Avenue, Milwaukee, WI 53226, USA
* Corresponding author.
E-mail address: spawar@mcw.edu

Facial Plast Surg Clin N Am 25 (2017) 263–270
http://dx.doi.org/10.1016/j.fsc.2016.12.009
1064-7406/17/© 2017 Elsevier Inc. All rights reserved.

guesswork needed to achieve a desired result. Similarly, computer modeling and simulation techniques have the potential to provide facial plastic surgeons with information that could aid in patient-specific surgical planning.

The accessibility to affordable, yet powerful hardware and software has fueled the emergence of very sophisticated computer modeling tools. Historically, modeling of biological hard and soft tissue modifications with endless variation and intrinsic tissue properties has been challenging. Medical imaging has been a key transformative technology in this regard because computed tomography (CT), magnetic resonance imaging (MRI), and ultrasound can now achieve extreme high levels of resolution and detail. This has facilitated the development of computations and simulations that were never previously possible. Additionally, commercially available software programs now provide tools to manipulate imaging data to simulate surgical modifications of specific anatomy.

Over the past several years, there have been an increasing number of studies using computer modeling tools to study the nose. This article reviews the specific modeling technologies of FEM and CFD, and their application to nasal surgery.

FINITE ELEMENT MODELING

FEM is a computational technique used to quantitatively study the biomechanics of a structure and provides a method to analyze structural stress, strain, and energy distributions on 3-dimensional (3D) structures.[2] The first multicomponent FEM of the nose incorporating bone, cartilage, and skin-soft tissue was reported by Manuel and colleagues.[3] Over the past several years, there have been an increasing number of studies applying FEM to various nasal constructs in addition to studying effects of specific rhinoplasty techniques.

Nasal Septum and Dorsum

Some of the initial studies applying FEM to the nose studied biomechanics of the septal L-strut.[4,5] Lee and colleagues[5] created several models by altering material properties of the septum and nasal tip support to determine the overall deformation and stress distribution in the L-strut. They found that the most consistent points of maximum stress were the bony-cartilaginous junction and the nasal spine, highlighting the importance of maintaining adequate cartilage support within the L-strut at these 2 locations. In more recent work, they further analyzed the caudal segment of the septal L-strut and highlighted the importance of maintaining at least 1 cm of septal cartilage width along the inferior portion of the L-strut, at

the junction with the anterior spine.[2] In another recent study, Tjoa and colleagues[6] used FEM to simulate wound healing forces and surgical maneuvers that may lead to the inverted V-deformity.

Cephalic Trim

FEM modeling of the nose has also been used to study effects of lower lateral cartilage resection on the overall mechanical stability of the nose and nasal cartilages. In an initial study, Oliaei and colleagues[7] developed an FEM of 3 different lower lateral cartilage widths, simulating differing amounts of cephalic resection. Using this model, they showed that there was no statistically significant decline in structural support of the cartilage when a minimum 6 mm width of lateral crus was maintained, suggesting that this width could potentially resist contractile forces related to postoperative scar tissue. In a more recent study, Leary and colleagues[8] applied FEM to study the potential impact of cephalic resection on the strength and stability of the lateral crus. They identified the common clinical problem of alar retraction after cephalic trim, and used FEM techniques to better understand the complex forces and factors that contribute to this complication. As they pointed out, objective analysis of rhinoplasty maneuvers is difficult to perform on patients due to the overall long period of time during which changes in nasal shape occur. Unfortunately, a limitation of current modeling techniques is the overall lack of experimental data to simulate these complex wound healing processes.

Nasal Tip Support

Other studies have applied FEM to investigate nasal tip dynamics and support.[3,7–11] Shamouelian and colleagues[10] examined relative contributions of 2 major tip support mechanisms: attachment between the lower and upper lateral cartilages (scroll region) and attachment of the medial crura to the caudal septum. Computer models were modified by removing various intercartilaginous connections to simulate various rhinoplasty maneuvers (transfixion and intercartilaginous incisions). Each model was then subjected to a nasal tip force to simulate nasal tip depression. Results of this modeling showed disruption of the medial crura attachment to the caudal septum had a greater impact on nasal tip support compared with disruption of the scroll region. In another study, FEM was used to study how columellar strut graft size, shape, and attachment to the medial crura affect nasal tip support.[11] Interestingly, suture placement to fixate the graft was found to be just as important as the strut size, with the most important point of fixation at the proximal or anterior portion of the columellar strut graft to the medial crura. In addition to studying cartilage biomechanics, FEM has also been used to evaluate the influence of columellar scar shape on the stress distribution within the tissue following an external rhinoplasty approach and supported the current practice of an inverted-V shaped columellar incision.[9]

COMPUTATIONAL FLUID DYNAMICS

While FEM provides an analysis of biomechanical forces within the nose, CFD enables a quantitative analysis of nasal airflow and offers several advantages over traditional objective measures. A myriad of tools have been used by clinicians to evaluate nasal airway obstruction (NAO) in the clinical setting. These include patient-reported questionnaires, physical examination maneuvers, and objective tests such as rhinomanometry[12] and acoustic rhinometry.[13] These tests do little to identify specific anatomic problems for correction, have low correlation with patient symptoms, and at best are capable of producing surgical failure rates as high as 37%.[14–20] This high failure rate has been attributed to the lack of a gold standard to diagnose the extent and cause of NAO, and lack of tools to aid surgeons in predicting surgical success accurately.

The complexity of the nasal airway is well suited to the creation of a computational tool to aid surgeons in the diagnosis and treatment of NAO. CFD is a well-established, powerful tool that can be used to model and analyze the biophysics of nasal airflow. With the availability of powerful bioengineering computer-aided design software, anatomically accurate 3D computational models can now be generated from CT or MRI data. CFD software can then be used to analyze these models and calculate various anatomic and physiologic measures, including nasal airflow, resistance, air conditioning, and wall shear stress. Furthermore, these 3D computational models can be modified to simulate surgical changes or perform virtual surgery. CFD tools can then be used to study the effects of these changes on nasal function and in the future, potentially aid in surgical planning and in predicting surgical outcomes.

CFD computations are based on known airflow dynamics and grounded in basic physical laws of fluid flow, such as the conservation of mass (continuity equation) and the conservation of momentum (Navier-Stokes equations). The latter is derived from Newton's second law applied to a fluid element.[21] In general, given a tube of any shape and the physical conditions producing airflow through the tube (called boundary conditions), the Navier-Stokes equations can be solved to obtain information about the flow such as velocity, pressure distribution, allocation of the flow to different regions within the tube, forces exerted on the walls (shear stress), how much the flow swirls (vorticity), and turbulence.[22] However, airflow in the nose is complicated by the irregular 3D shape of the nasal cavity, areas of marked constriction, abrupt changes in direction of airflow, and areas in which the dimensions of the airway are under muscular and vascular control. These factors impose some limitations on the interpretation of nasal resistance measurements because the nasal airway cavity cannot be represented as an ideal tube by the simplest physical laws of fluid flow.

Computational Fluid Dynamics Workflow

The process of developing a patient-specific CFD model begins with raw CT or MRI data, which then goes through a process of segmentation to create an initial 3D model using medical imaging software, such as Mimics (Materialise, Plymouth, MI, USA) (**Fig. 1**). To solve the equations that govern fluid flow, each 3D nasal model must be divided into a large number of small cells in which air velocity and pressure can be defined. This is accomplished by creating a mesh with approximately 4 million tetrahedral cells using ICEM-CFD (ANSYS Inc, Canonsburg, PA, USA). Airflow simulations for flow rates corresponding to normal resting breathing are conducted using Fluent (ANSYS Inc, Canonsburg, PA, USA). The following boundary conditions are often used to determine the steady-state airflow field: (1) a wall condition (zero velocity, stationary wall assumed) at the airway walls, (2) a pressure-inlet condition at the nostrils with gauge pressure set to 0, and (3) a pressure-outlet condition at the outlet with gauge pressure set to a negative value in pascals that generates the target steady state inhalation rate of 15.0 L/min. This flow rate represents a healthy adult breathing at rest.[23] Additional details on the differential equations, computational algorithms, and air physical properties used can be found in previous publications.[24] Figures, printouts, diagrams, and other visualizations of CFD model results can be made using the visualization software package Fieldview (Intelligent Light, Lyndhurst, NJ, USA), as well as the with the visualization capabilities within Fluent.

Although CFD technology has become increasingly available, until recently it was still a time-intensive endeavor to create individual CFD models. Therefore, previous studies used only small cohorts (fewer than 5 subjects) with a focus more on feasibility rather than clinical correlation. Also, many of

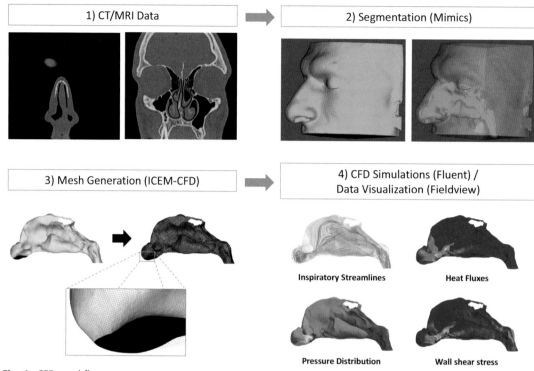

Fig. 1. CFD workflow.

these studies did not have corroborating postsurgical data for comparisons. Modeling methods have now evolved from years-long efforts to create a single model from sparse image data in the 1990s to the ability to create a model from high-resolution CT scans and run the CFD simulations within days. These methods are now enabling human CFD studies with larger cohorts with statistical power.

Computational Fluid Dynamics and Nasal Airway Obstruction

The application of CFD to the study of NAO and functional nasal surgery is a novel use of this technology and has the potential to alter the landscape of functional nasal surgery. Early studies demonstrated the ability of CFD to accurately describe biophysics of nasal airflow and the relationship between form and function, including investigation of the aerodynamic consequences of abnormal nasal anatomy,[25–27] surgery,[24,28–33] or creation of template models of healthy nasal anatomy.[34,35] The initial studies formed the basis for the more recent CFD investigations with larger cohort sizes.

The next stage of CFD research sought to correlate CFD variables with subjective symptoms of nasal obstruction as reported on the Nasal Obstruction Symptom Evaluation (NOSE) scale[36] or visual analog scales.[37] Recent publications

have found linear correlations between patient-reported symptoms and several CFD variables, including[38,39]

1. Unilateral airflow
2. Airflow partition (distribution of airflow between left and right sides of the nose)
3. Unilateral heat flux
4. Nasal resistance ratio (unilateral nasal airway resistance as a fraction of bilateral nasal resistance)
5. Unilateral mucosal surface area where heat flux is greater than 50 W/m^2.

These correlations have implications for functional analysis of the nose and targeting CFD parameters through virtual surgery. Interestingly, heat flux measures have received special focus because a growing body of literature suggests that the feeling of nasal patency has a better correlation with the cooling effect that inspired air has on nasal mucosa than with airflow or nasal resistance.[40,41] The surface area where heat flux exceeds 50 W/m^2 is a measure of the surface area of nasal mucosa stimulated by mucosal cooling and is currently being investigated as a parameter that may have some significance to patient perception of nasal obstruction. In a recent study, virtual surgery was used to compare the impact of total inferior turbinectomy (TIT) versus total middle turbinectomy (TMT) on nasal resistance and nasal air conditioning.[42] The investigators reported that TIT reduced nasal resistance to a greater extent but also was associated with a greater reduction in the nasal humidification capacity compared with TMT. Interestingly, the surface area stimulated by mucosal cooling (ie, the surface area where heat flux exceeds 50 W/m^2) decreased after TIT. The investigators speculated that this reduction in mucosal cooling after TIT may explain the paradoxical sensation of nasal obstruction in empty nose syndrome patients.

Computational Fluid Dynamics and Virtual Nasal Surgery

Preliminary research has demonstrated the potential for CFD virtual surgery simulations to predict results of in vivo real surgery.[43] An initial study used a single patient model to create 3 virtual surgery models that were then compared with an actual postsurgical model.[44] Subsequent work used a larger cohort to compare CFD variables in presurgery, virtual surgery, and postsurgery models of 10 NAO subjects.[43] Using patient-specific models, this type of computational analysis has the potential to provide important information regarding the efficacy of specific techniques for a given patient. The surgical effect can be estimated by comparing changes in CFD variables in virtual surgery models built from presurgery imaging to normative CFD data derived from healthy subjects without NAO.

The effect of individual surgical maneuvers on CFD parameters can be analyzed in isolation and in various combinations. One study used virtual surgery techniques to quantify effects of individual components of nasal airway surgery, including septoplasty, bilateral turbinate reduction, and nasal valve repair in a single patient.[45] Actual presurgery and postsurgery models were created from a patient who underwent these procedures and the effects of each component of the surgery were isolated. In this case, most of the reduction in nasal resistance was attributed to the septoplasty and inferior turbinate reduction, whereas the contribution of the nasal valve repair was found to be relatively less. In another study, Shadfar and colleagues[46] performed various flare suture techniques and spreader grafts on a cadaver head and then used CFD models to compare the effects of these techniques on nasal resistance, nasal airflow, and nasal airflow partitioning. They found that the medial and modified flare suture techniques alone provided the greatest improvement in nasal airflow and nasal resistance compared with spreader grafts alone or in combination with flare sutures. Although very preliminary, the results of this CFD analysis introduce the concept that flare sutures alone could be a better technique for addressing the internal nasal valve as opposed to the more traditional cartilage grafting techniques that many surgeons currently use.[46]

One of the current challenges for surgeons performing functional nasal surgery is deciding which nasal structures should be surgically altered to provide the most relief from symptoms. The nasal septum, inferior turbinates, and nasal valve region are the areas typically targeted during functional nasal surgery. On one end of the spectrum, extensive surgery involving all of these structures would yield the largest nasal airway but possibly at the expense of other nasal functions, including air heating, humidification, and filtration. On the other end of the spectrum, minimally invasive surgery may not relieve symptoms but is often preferred due to minimized surgical risks such as infection, wound healing problems, and empty nose syndrome.[47,48] The tradeoff between more extensive surgery with potentially more benefits to patients or less surgery with reduced costs and lower risks, motivates development of a computational tool for surgical planning.

Given the current state of CFD technology and knowledge base, the potential exists to identify the optimal surgical procedures for each individual patient through virtual surgery CFD manipulation of preoperative nasal models. By combining these virtual surgery techniques with CFD variables that have been shown to correlate with patient-reported symptoms, it will ultimately be possible to prospectively predict which nasal procedures will have the potential to bring abnormal CFD variables into the normative range and likely yield the best patient outcome (**Fig. 2**).

LIMITATIONS OF COMPUTATIONAL MODELING

Although FEM and CFD applications for nasal surgery are certainly promising, there are several inherent limitations in the current state of this technology[7]:

1. Modeling of complex structures, such as the nose, is challenging.
2. Material properties of most biological materials are unknown and, generally, nonlinear and anisotropic.
3. Most CFD models assume rigid walls and thus do not account for nasal valve collapse.
4. User-friendly software applications are not yet available.

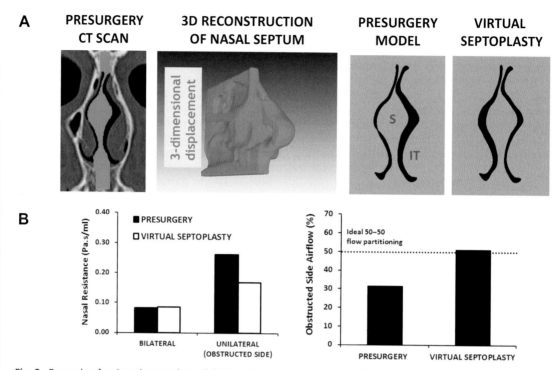

Fig. 2. Example of a virtual septoplasty. (*A*) Virtual septoplasty can be performed using 3D deformation software. (*B*) Virtual septoplasty decreased nasal resistance on the obstructed side and achieved a 50%-50% flow partitioning between the left and right cavities.

Both FEM and CFD techniques use several assumptions to simplify the computational process. In general, mechanical properties in FEM are assumed to be linearly elastic and isotropic, although, in reality, biologic tissues are viscoelastic and anisotropic.[3] In the case of CFD, simulations use a fixed wall model, which cannot account for compliance of the nasal soft tissues in the presence of negative pressure. In addition, these models assume that complete airflow occurs through the nose only, although, in reality, patients with varying degrees of NAO will breathe through the mouth, potentially altering the true airflow characteristics in the nose. Another modeling challenge is that each computational model represents the nasal anatomy at a specific point in time. Although major structural features will generally be preserved across models, the dynamic nature of the nasal mucosa (ie, nasal cycling) can vary between models of the same patient and potentially influence direct comparisons.[49] This has the potential to become problematic when applying CFD techniques to the relatively narrow nasal passages, where only a few millimeters of mucosal swelling can result in significant airflow changes.[50] In addition, although virtual surgery can be done on a static model, the unpredictable and dynamic nature of patient healing can ultimately limit the

predictive capability of the model. Additionally, although virtual surgery models can come close to mirroring actual postsurgical models, there are still limitations in translating actual surgical maneuvers to a 3D computer model.[43] Currently, virtual surgery is performed by manually editing multiple 2D cross-sections to mimic 3D changes. This is a crude and labor-intensive method that does not accurately substitute the experience or findings during actual surgery.

Aside from the inherent limitations in the models themselves, there are important practical considerations. Although CFD software applications have become more widely available and accessible, they remain costly and are often cumbersome to use. Also, the current workflow to create computational models and run various simulations is time consuming and requires a level of technical expertise that is not available to most surgeons.

SUMMARY

The future of computer modeling techniques, such as FEM and CFD, and their applications in functional nasal surgery are promising. These technologies will have educational applications in teaching complex concepts in nasal anatomy and physiology to students and surgeons. There is no question that surgeon experience, technical skills, and knowledge will remain the basis for excellent patient care and optimal surgical outcomes. However, these modeling technologies have the potential to equip rhinoplasty surgeons with information to truly individualize the care they provide and achieve the best possible outcomes for patients.

REFERENCES

1. Mathog RH, Leonard M, Bevis R. Surgical correction of maxillary hypoplasia. Arch Otolaryngol 1979; 105(7):399–403.

2. Lee J-S, Lee DC, Ha D-H, et al. Redefining the septal L-strut in septal surgery. PLoS One 2015; 10(3):e0119996.

3. Manuel CT, Leary R, Protsenko DE, et al. Nasal tip support: a finite element analysis of the role of the caudal septum during tip depression. Laryngoscope 2014;124(3):649–54.

4. Mau T, Mau S-T, Kim DW. Cadaveric and engineering analysis of the septal L-strut. Laryngoscope 2007;117(11):1902–6.

5. Lee SJ, Liong K, Tse KM, et al. Biomechanics of the deformity of septal L-Struts. Laryngoscope 2010; 120(8):1508–15.

6. Tjoa T, Manuel CT, Leary RP, et al. A finite element model to simulate formation of the inverted-V deformity. JAMA Facial Plast Surg 2016;18(2):136–43.

7. Oliaei S, Manuel C, Protsenko D, et al. Mechanical analysis of the effects of cephalic trim on lower lateral cartilage stability. Arch Facial Plast Surg 2012;14(1):27–30.

8. Leary RP, Manuel CT, Shamouelian D, et al. Finite element model analysis of cephalic trim on nasal tip stability. JAMA Facial Plast Surg 2015;17(6): 413–20.

9. Gizzi A, Cherubini C, Pomella N, et al. Computational modeling and stress analysis of columellar biomechanics. J Mech Behav Biomed Mater 2012; 15:46–58.

10. Shamouelian D, Leary RP, Manuel CT, et al. Rethinking nasal tip support: a finite element analysis. Laryngoscope 2015;125(2):326–30.

11. Gandy JR, Manuel CT, Leary RP, et al. Quantifying optimal columellar strut dimensions for nasal tip stabilization after rhinoplasty via finite element analysis. JAMA Facial Plast Surg 2016;18(3):194–200.

12. Cole P. Nasal airflow resistance: a survey of 2500 assessments. Am J Rhinol 1997;11(6):415–20.

13. Hilberg O, Jackson AC, Swift DL, et al. Acoustic rhinometry: evaluation of nasal cavity geometry by acoustic reflection. J Appl Physiol (1985) 1989;66(1): 295–303.

14. André RF, D'Souza AR, Kunst HP, et al. Sub-alar batten grafts as treatment for nasal valve incompetence; description of technique and functional evaluation. Rhinology 2006;44(2):118–22.

15. Illum P. Septoplasty and compensatory inferior turbinate hypertrophy: long-term results after randomized turbinoplasty. Eur Arch Otorhinolaryngol 1997; 254(Suppl 1):S89–92.

16. Samad I, Stevens HE, Maloney A. The efficacy of nasal septal surgery. J Otolaryngol 1992;21(2): 88–91.

17. Singh A, Patel N, Kenyon G, et al. Is there objective evidence that septal surgery improves nasal airflow? J Laryngol Otol 2006;120(11):916–20.

18. Rhee JS, McMullin BT. Measuring outcomes in facial plastic surgery: a decade of progress. Curr Opin Otolaryngol Head Neck Surg 2008;16(4):387–93.

19. Pawar SS, Garcia GJM, Kimbell JS, et al. Objective measures in aesthetic and functional nasal surgery: perspectives on nasal form and function. Facial Plast Surg 2010;26(4):320–7.

20. André RF, Vuyk HD, Ahmed A, et al. Correlation between subjective and objective evaluation of the nasal airway. A systematic review of the highest level of evidence. Clin Otolaryngol 2009;34(6):518–25.

21. White FM. Fluid mechanics. New York: McGraw-Hill; 2008.

22. Batchelor GK. An introduction to fluid dynamics. Cambridge (UK): Cambridge University Press; 1973.

23. Garcia GJM, Schroeter JD, Segal RA, et al. Dosimetry of nasal uptake of water-soluble and reactive gases: a first study of interhuman variability. Inhal Toxicol 2009;21(7):607–18.

24. Garcia GJM, Bailie N, Martins DA, et al. Atrophic rhinitis: a CFD study of air conditioning in the nasal cavity. J Appl Physiol (1985) 2007;103(3):1082–92.

25. Zhu JH, Lee HP, Lim KM, et al. Inspirational airflow patterns in deviated noses: a numerical study. Comput Methods Biomech Biomed Engin 2013;16(12): 1298–306.

26. Liu T, Han D, Wang J, et al. Effects of septal deviation on the airflow characteristics: using computational fluid dynamics models. Acta Otolaryngol 2012;132(3):290–8.

27. Li L, Han D, Zhang L, et al. Aerodynamic investigation of the correlation between nasal septal deviation and chronic rhinosinusitis. Laryngoscope 2012; 122(9):1915–9.

28. Chen XB, Lee HP, Chong VFH, et al. Assessment of septal deviation effects on nasal air flow: a computational fluid dynamics model. Laryngoscope 2009; 119(9):1730–6.

29. Wang T, Mu X, Deng J, et al. Investigation on the structure of nasal cavity and its airflow field in Crouzon syndrome. J Craniofac Surg 2011;22(1):166–72.

30. Iwasaki T, Saitoh I, Takemoto Y, et al. Improvement of nasal airway ventilation after rapid maxillary expansion evaluated with computational fluid

dynamics. Am J Orthod Dentofacial Orthop 2012; 141(3):269–78.

31. Ozlugedik S, Nakiboglu G, Sert C, et al. Numerical study of the aerodynamic effects of septoplasty and partial lateral turbinectomy. Laryngoscope 2008;118(2):330–4.

32. Chen XB, Leong SC, Lee HP, et al. Aerodynamic effects of inferior turbinate surgery on nasal airflow–a computational fluid dynamics model. Rhinology 2010;48(4):394–400.

33. Lindemann J, Brambs H-J, Keck T, et al. Numerical simulation of intranasal airflow after radical sinus surgery. Am J Otolaryngol 2005;26(3):175–80.

34. Gambaruto AM, Taylor DJ, Doorly DJ. Decomposition and description of the nasal cavity form. Ann Biomed Eng 2012;40(5):1142–59.

35. Liu Y, Johnson MR, Matida EA, et al. Creation of a standardized geometry of the human nasal cavity. J Appl Physiol (1985) 2009;106(3):784–95.

36. Stewart MG, Smith TL, Weaver EM, et al. Outcomes after nasal septoplasty: results from the Nasal Obstruction Septoplasty Effectiveness (NOSE) study. Otolaryngol Head Neck Surg 2004;130(3):283–90.

37. Rhee JS, Sullivan CD, Frank DO, et al. A systematic review of patient-reported nasal obstruction scores: defining normative and symptomatic ranges in surgical patients. JAMA Facial Plast Surg 2014;16(3):219–25 [quiz: 232].

38. Kimbell JS, Frank DO, Laud P, et al. Changes in nasal airflow and heat transfer correlate with symptom improvement after surgery for nasal obstruction. J Biomech 2013;46(15):2634–43.

39. Sullivan CD, Garcia GJM, Frank-Ito DO, et al. Perception of better nasal patency correlates with increased mucosal cooling after surgery for nasal obstruction. Otolaryngol Head Neck Surg 2014; 150(1):139–47.

40. Zhao K, Blacker K, Luo Y, et al. Perceiving nasal patency through mucosal cooling rather than air temperature or nasal resistance. PLoS One 2011; 6(10):e24618.

41. Eccles R, Jones AS. The effect of menthol on nasal resistance to air flow. J Laryngol Otol 1983;97(8):705–9.

42. Dayal A, Rhee JS, Garcia GJM. Impact of middle versus inferior total turbinectomy on nasal aerodynamics. Otolaryngol Head Neck Surg 2016;155(3):518–25.

43. Frank-Ito DO, Kimbell JS, Laud P, et al. Predicting postsurgery nasal physiology with computational modeling: current challenges and limitations. Otolaryngol Head Neck Surg 2014;151(5):751–9.

44. Rhee JS, Pawar SS, Garcia GJM, et al. Toward personalized nasal surgery using computational fluid dynamics. Arch Facial Plast Surg 2011;13(5):305–10.

45. Rhee JS, Cannon DE, Frank DO, et al. Role of virtual surgery in preoperative planning: assessing the individual components of functional nasal airway surgery. Arch Facial Plast Surg 2012;14(5):354–9.

46. Shadfar S, Shockley WW, Fleischman GM, et al. Characterization of postoperative changes in nasal airflow using a cadaveric computational fluid dynamics model: supporting the internal nasal valve. JAMA Facial Plast Surg 2014;16(5):319–27.

47. Houser SM. Empty nose syndrome associated with middle turbinate resection. Otolaryngol Head Neck Surg 2006;135(6):972–3.

48. Moore EJ, Kern EB. Atrophic rhinitis: a review of 242 cases. Am J Rhinol 2001;15(6):355–61.

49. Patel RG, Garcia GJM, Frank-Ito DO, et al. Simulating the nasal cycle with computational fluid dynamics. Otolaryngol Head Neck Surg 2015;152(2):353–60.

50. Quine SM, Aitken PM, Eccles R. Effect of submucosal diathermy to the inferior turbinates on unilateral and total nasal airflow in patients with rhinitis. Acta Otolaryngol 2009;119(8):911–5.

Index

Note: Page numbers of article titles are in **boldface** type.

A

Abscess, of nasal septum, in children, 217

Acellular dermis grafts, for dorsal correction, in saddle deformity, 244, 247, 249

Acoustic rhinometry, for ENV collapse, 186
  for functional rhinoplasty, 157
  for saddle deformity, 240

Adjunct medications, for rhinoplasty, with osteotomies, 202–203

Airflow, assessment of dynamics of. See *Computational fluid dynamics (CFD).*
  in ENV physiology, 183, 185
  in INV compromise, 197
  in saddle deformity repair, 243, 248
  with rhinoplasty, 195–196
    complications of, 252–253
    primary vs. secondary, in children, 218

Airway obstruction. See *Nasal airway obstruction (NAO).*

Alar base, in cleft nasal deformity repair, unilateral, 225–226
  in revision rhinoplasty, 257–259
  in secondary cleft septorhinoplasty, 231–232, 235

Alar batten grafts, for ENV collapse, 187–190, 192, 198
  in revision rhinoplasty, 258–259

Alar groove, in ENV anatomy, 179–180, 198

Alar lobule, in ENV anatomy, 179–180
  in functional rhinoplasty, anatomy of, 143, 146–147
    columella-to-lobule ratio, 152, 154

Alar rim, in ENV anatomy, 180, 185
  in secondary cleft septorhinoplasty, 231–232, 235

Alar rim grafts, for ENV collapse, 191–192, 198
  in secondary cleft septorhinoplasty, 232, 235–236

Alar strut grafts, in secondary cleft septorhinoplasty, 235

Alar turn-in flap, in secondary cleft septorhinoplasty, 235

Alloderm, for dorsal correction, in saddle deformity, 244, 247, 249

Allografts, for dorsal correction, in saddle deformity, 244–246

Alveolar bone grafts, in secondary cleft septorhinoplasty, 227, 231–233

Anesthesia, for nasal septal fractures reduction, in children, 216–217
  for rhinoplasty, with osteotomies, 202

Animal studies, of pediatric rhinoplasty, 212

Anterior septal reconstruction (ASR), for anterocaudal deviation, intraoperative images, 165–168
    patient outcomes, 167–168
    repair vs., 164–165
    technique for, 166–168
  modified extracorporeal resection as, in septoplasty, 165–168

Anterocaudal septal deviation, ENV collapse and, 185
  septoplasty for, challenges, 164–165
    description of planes, 164
    management strategies, 164–165
    reconstruction technique, 165–168

Antihistamines, for inferior turbinate hypertrophy, 173–174

Arterial blood supply, to inferior turbinate, 172
  to nose, 147–150

ASR. See *Anterior septal reconstruction (ASR).*

Autologous grafts, for dorsal correction, in saddle deformity, 244–248
    comparison of, 249

Axis, short vs. long, in ENV anatomy, 180, 190

B

Batten grafts, alar, for ENV collapse, 187–190, 192, 198
    in revision rhinoplasty, 258–259
    in saddle deformity repair, 243, 245, 248

Bernoulli principle, in ENV physiology, 183

Biofeedback, for ENV collapse, 186

Bleeding, with rhinoplasty, medications to reduce, 202–203

Blood supply, in functional rhinoplasty, 147–150
    to external nose, 148–149
    to inferior turbinate, 172
    to left nasal septum, 148, 150
    to right lateral nasal wall, 148, 150

Bolsters, in cleft lip nasal deformity repair, 218

Bone grafts, alveolar, in secondary cleft septorhinoplasty, 227, 231–233
  for dorsal correction, in saddle deformity, 244, 247
    split calvarial, 246, 249

Bone/bony pyramid, of nose, fracture patterns of, in children, 215–216
  growth and development of, in infants, 212–213
  in cleft nasal deformity repair, bilateral, 226–227
  in functional rhinoplasty, anatomy of, 142
    in infants, 202
    septal, 161–162, 166

Facial Plast Surg Clin N Am 25 (2017) 271–282
http://dx.doi.org/10.1016/S1064-7406(17)30010-X
1064-7406/17